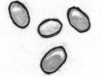

Why

Is

Brian

So

Fat?

Why Is Brian So Fat?

By Gary Solomon, PhD

Illustrated by Lynne Adamson

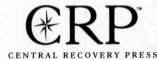

CENTRAL RECOVERY PRESS

CENTRAL RECOVERY PRESS

Central Recovery Press (CRP) is committed to publishing exceptional materials addressing addiction treatment, recovery, and behavioral healthcare topics, including original and quality books, audio/visual communications, and web-based new media. Through a diverse selection of titles, we seek to contribute a broad range of unique resources for professionals, recovering individuals and their families, and the general public.

For more information, visit www.centralrecoverypress.com.

Central Recovery Press, Las Vegas, NV 89129

Publisher: Central Recovery Press
             3321 N. Buffalo Drive
             Las Vegas, NV 89129

17 16 15 14 13 12   1 2 3 4 5

ISBN-13: 978-1-936290-74-1 (paper)
ISBN-10: 1-936290-74-X
ISBN-13: 978-1-936290-76-5 (e-book)

Cover design and illustrations by Lynne Adamson
Interior design and layout by Sara Streifel, Think Creative Design

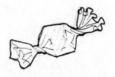

To my sister, Marlene, though you grew up just down the hall from me, I never really knew you. I know what I went through; you must have gone through the same thing.

We never had much of a chance at life. I made it; you did not.

Marlene, this one's for you.

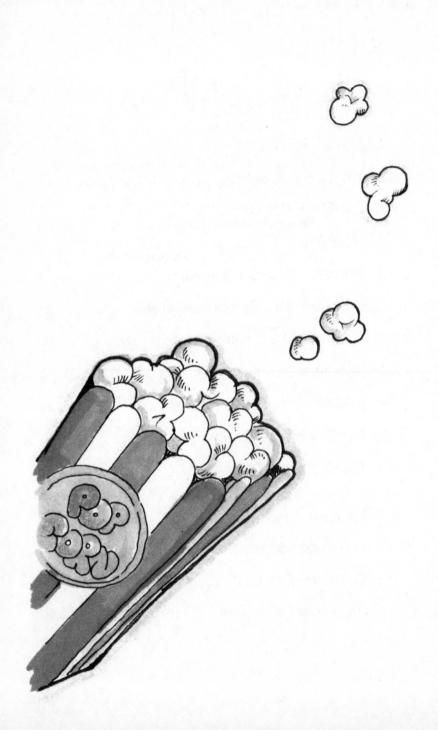

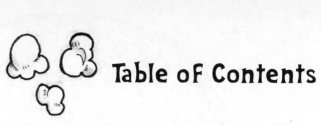

Table of Contents

Introduction...i

1. Almost All "A"s...1

2. What's For Dinner?.................................9

3. The Stash Drawer...................................17

4. Trouble..27

5. There's a New Kid in Town................39

6. If It's Not One Thing, It's Another......47

7. Meet the Armstrongs............................55

8. Yesterday and Today.............................67

9. Busted...79

10 The Day of the Big Exam....................87

11. Thank You Ms. Diaz...............................101

Epilogue...117

Activity Guide and Discussion Questions...........118

Things You Can Do to Stay Healthy..............124

Resources For Kids and Parents.....................126

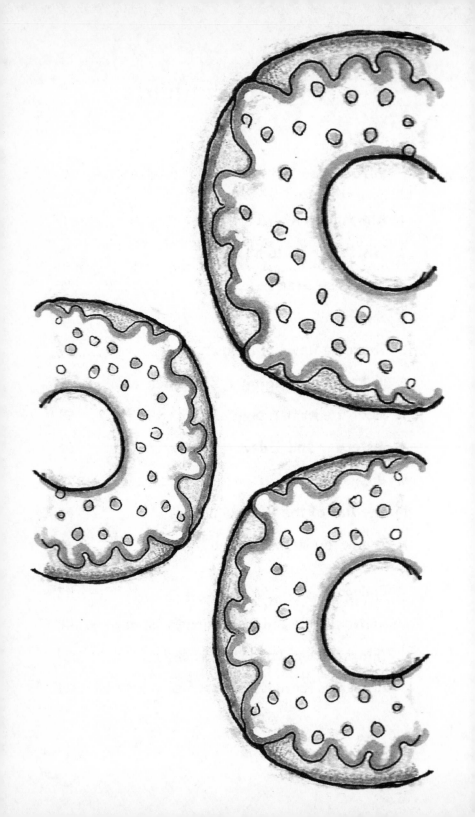

Introduction

This is a story about Brian. Brian is like most children and yet, he is different from a lot of children. He's not tall like a basketball player or strong like a football player or fast like a runner. No, he doesn't have three heads and he's not one of those kids who can play a musical instrument. Brian, well, how should I say this? To be totally honest, Brian is just fat. I could say that he is pleasingly plump or just going through a stage or heavyset or lots of other descriptions that would apply to Brian, but the truth is, he's fat.

To me it's important for everyone to know why Brian is fat. He's fat because he eats too much. And he eats too much because that's how he deals with his feelings. Brian has lots of feelings about his family, and many of those feelings he's not even aware of having. So this story is also about Brian's family: Charlotte, his mother; Marshall, his father; and Madison, his sister.

Brian's family lives in the same way most families do. Oh, maybe they are better off than some, but not as well off as others. But basically they're the same as every other family, at least that's the way it seems. Maybe after reading this story about them, you will see what's different about Brian and his family and you will understand why Brian is so fat.

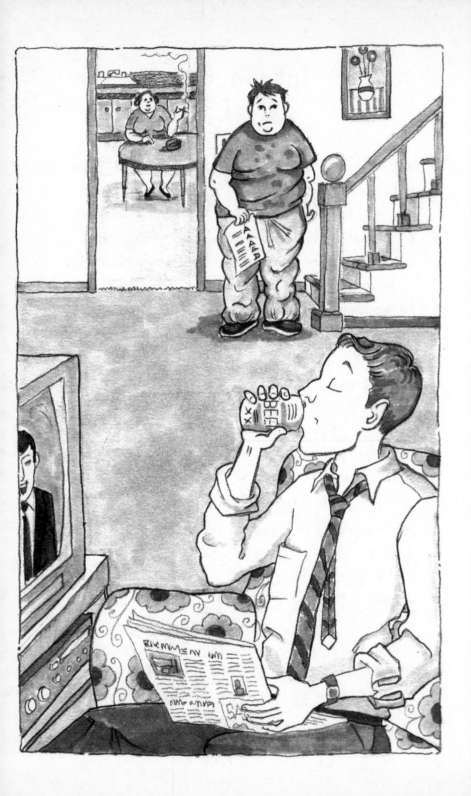

Almost All "A"s

"Mom, Mom, Dad's home," yelled Brian as he leaped away from the window where he'd been standing. Brian was excited because today he'd received his report card. Straight "A"s. Well, almost. There was that one little "D" he got in physical education, but that didn't ruin his excitement. Brian was used to getting a "D" in physical education, and he wasn't going to let that grade ruin an otherwise perfect report card. *All "A"s,* he thought as he ran to the door to greet his father, who was coming home from work. *All "A"s!*

The "A"s were special for Brian. Special, because it meant that he got extra attention. He didn't get much attention except at report card time, and a twelve-and-a-half-year-old likes attention sometimes, even if it's just for a stupid old report card that his sister Madison couldn't care less about.

"Why do you worry so much about that stuff?" Madison would ask. "All you ever do is play those lame video games. You know you wouldn't be so fat if you'd do something other than sit around all day. You could exercise like I do."

Madison was always exercising, and if she wasn't exercising she was running, and if she wasn't running she was jumping, and if she wasn't jumping she was riding her bike. In fact, Madison never sat still. *But that is no concern of mine,* Brian thought, *because today is my day.* Today is a day of straight "A"s. Well, almost.

Brian ran with a waddle around the overstuffed couch to the steps that led down the hallway to the front door of the house. Just at the moment when Brian was taking his second step into the hallway, he heard his mother yell from the kitchen, "Brian, get your dad a beer." *Why do I always have to get Dad a beer?* he thought.

"Okay," he yelled. He turned as quickly as his body would allow and ran down the hallway to the door that led into the garage where the beer was kept in a refrigerator filled with beer and diet colas. In the freezer was container after container of ice cream. Brian and his mom loved ice cream.

Brian thought to himself, *I hate the smell of this stuff. How can Dad stand to drink this junk?* He remembered Madison told him that sometimes she would go into the fridge and take out a bottle of beer. She said she kind of liked the "buzz" it gave her.

Brian remembered the time he caught Madison drinking a beer and he swore on his life he wouldn't tell.

"Dad will kill me. I won't be able to go out of the house for a year. Please, please," Madison begged. "Please don't tell on me."

Brian thought for a minute and then replied, "Well, okay, but you have to give me your dessert from your lunch every day for a week." Madison never ate the desserts in her lunch anyway. She would throw them away instead of giving them to Brian just to make him mad.

So, because of the deal they made, Brian never said a word to Dad or anyone else.

Even though Brian didn't like the smell of beer, he had to admit that Dad always enjoyed his beer and after about three or four bottles of the stuff he seemed to calm down, especially after what his dad called a "long, hard, miserable day at work." *Dad works hard*, Brian thought. *Sometimes he works all weekend long. Sometimes he even comes home after I go to bed. I guess when you work that hard you must need a drink. But why does Madison drink it?* Brian wondered. *Why does she like it?*

He grabbed the beer and ran back to the door as fast as he could.

He heard the sound of a key going into the lock as he stood with the beer in his hand, smiling from ear to ear. *Dad is going to be so proud of me. Another great report card!*

The large wooden door opened and Marshall, Brian's father, stepped inside the house. Brian was always a little amazed at how his father could take just one giant step and end up in the house. Marshall was a big man, tall and lean, with great big hands and lanky, long legs.

"Thanks, Bri Bri," his dad said with a smile. "You're a good man." His dad had called him "Bri Bri" ever since Brian could remember. "Thanks for the beer. I really need it today."

He says that all the time, Brian thought.

"It's been another long, hard, miserable ...." Brian sighed and turned off the rest of the sentence in his head.

"Dad, Dad, guess what? I got my report card and ..."

"Not now, Bri Bri. I need some time to put my feet up and have this beer. Give me a little time. Have you seen the paper? Anybody seen the paper?" he yelled, not giving Brian a chance to answer.

"Here it is, Dad," Madison said, stopping her exercising for a minute. "I put it on the table. I was using the couch for some of my stretching and forgot to put it back. Sorry."

"That's okay," her dad said, "just so it's here."

Oh great. That's terrific, Brian grumbled to himself.

He knew if his dad didn't take the time to read his report card now he surely wouldn't want to see it later. By the time his dad had a second beer, he wasn't much interested in anything. Brian had to tell him now.

"But Dad," Brian yelled. "I got my report card. I got straight 'A's. Don't you want to see it?"

"Now Brian," his dad said with an annoyed tone in his voice. "You get the same report card all the time. I'll bet you got that 'D' in PE again, didn't you?"

"Well . . . yes," Brian said, his eyes held tightly open, a quiver in his voice.

"My gosh, Brian! Can't you ever do any better than that? It's no wonder you get 'D's. You can't do anything in PE, can you? You're never going to be able to play any sports if you don't get rid of some of that fat."

"Marshall," Brian's mother interrupted as she walked out of the kitchen and into the living room. "You know how sensitive Brian is about his weight. Leave him alone. He can't help it if he's fat. Some kids are just fat. That's all."

"Oh, Charlotte," Marshall shouted. "Why don't you stay out of this? No one was talking to you anyway. We wouldn't have this problem if you would stop feeding him so much."

Brian had not moved an inch. Marshall turned his head to watch Madison still doing her exercises.

"Why don't you take your sister as an example and work out a little?" Brian shook his head up and down, but didn't say a word. Marshall threw up his hands in disgust. "Bri Bri, leave me alone for a while. I'll look at your report card later. It's been one of those days, if you know what I mean."

Brian's dad walked into the living room, never looking back. He grabbed the paper off the table, pulled at his tie and gave it a couple of hard yanks. He sank down into the couch that sat right in front of the television, took a sip of his beer, and let out a sigh. He let out a laugh and began his nightly job of reading the paper and complaining about the news of the day.

Brian held back the tears. "I wanted a special day and look what I got," he mumbled to himself. *Oh well, I guess he does work hard and he's right,* Brian thought. *I do need to lose some weight.* He stood at the foot of the steps for a moment and watched his dad read the paper and drink his beer. He shrugged his shoulders and began walking toward the kitchen where his mother was sitting at the table staring off into nowhere with a lit cigarette in her hand.

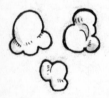

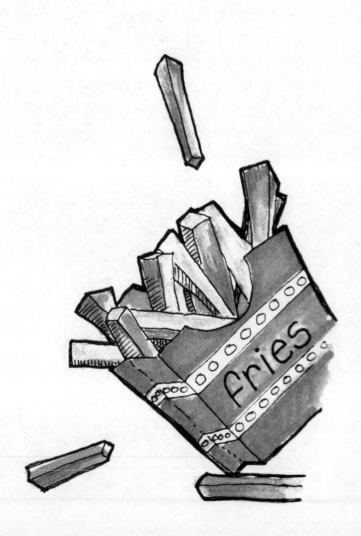

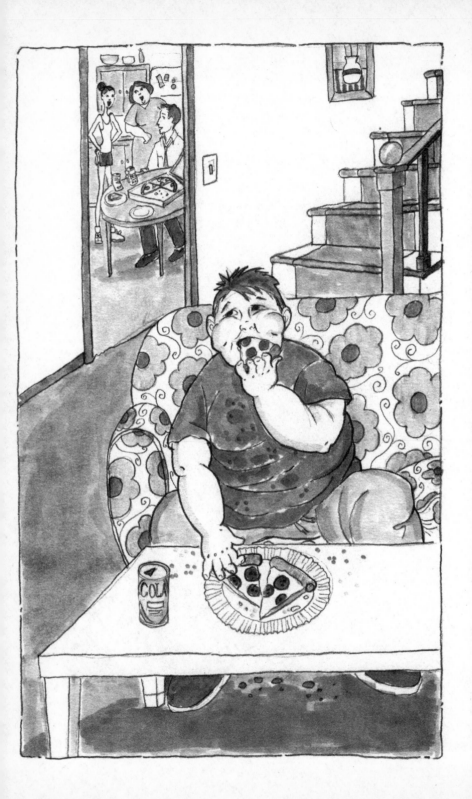

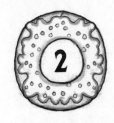

What's For Dinner?

"When's the pizza going to get here?" Brian yelled. "I'm starving." Before his mother had a chance to answer, Brian yelled again, "Can I have a cupcake before the pizza comes? I'm starving. I can't wait." He hadn't realized he was so hungry.

"Pizza's here," Charlotte barked. "Come on; hurry up before it gets cold."

Brian shoved the last bite of the cupcake down his throat. *Much better,* he thought. Brian's mom didn't mind that Brian had the cupcake because she felt so bad about the way his dad had treated him. She also knew how quickly food could soothe hurt feelings. Charlotte had put on a lot of weight in the past ten years. Food offered her a bit of happiness.

"Don't mind your dad. You know how he gets when he comes home from work. I barely talk to him much myself these days. Marriage is like that, you know, Brian. It seems after a while there's not much to say. Plus, I don't like talking to him when he's been working as much as he has been these last few years. And his drinking seems to have gotten worse. I don't think I'll stay with your father when you kids are grown. If it weren't for you and Madison, I don't think your father and I would be together at all. But that's life. 'You gotta stay together for the kids whether you like it or not.' At least that's what my mom used to say."

I'll never be that way when I get married, Brian thought to himself. *It's going to be different for me. My dad just doesn't know how to be nice to Mom.*

Just as the cupcake went kerplunk in his stomach, Brian saw his sister come dancing into the kitchen. Madison had on blue shorts and a yellow tank top with socks and sneakers to match. Her hair was pulled into a tight knot. She had just finished her aerobic workout.

"What's for dinner?" she asked in a let's-get-it-over-with tone of voice.

"Pizza," Brian replied without a moment's pause. His mom usually either nuked some kind of frozen dinner in the microwave or had some fast food delivered. Rarely did she actually cook a meal.

"Pizza," Madison whined. "Yuck!" she exclaimed. "Mom, I'm going to have some yogurt instead, and then I'm going over to MaryAnn's to practice my cheerleading. All this junk food makes me feel like a cow. I don't like it, anyway."

"Madison," her mother snapped back at her, "don't talk about food like that. You don't have to eat so much that you feel like a cow. Just eat some of the dinner. What about all the children all over the world who are starving? What about them?" Charlotte paused for a moment while she put the paper plates on the table. "And another thing, can't you ever have MaryAnn over to our house to practice your cheerleading? Why do you always have to go over to her house?"

"Mom, you know," she took a passing glance at her dad lying on the couch. "I just like it better over there. Please?" Her mom ignored Madison's glance at the couch and went on with what she had been doing.

Brian thought, *boy is she crazy. Pizza is the best kind of stuff in the world.* A mischievous grin peeked out under his chubby cheeks. *If she eats yogurt then there will be that much more pizza for me.*

"Madison," her mother continued, "a growing girl doesn't live on yogurt alone, you know."

"But Mom," Madison moaned. At that moment Brian's father strolled into the kitchen.

"What's going on in here? What's all this ruckus about? Why isn't everybody sitting down to eat? Brian,

I'm surprised you haven't started eating already. My goodness, sometimes I think if I don't get in here fast enough you'll have eaten everything all up. A man's got to be quick on his feet with old Bri Bri around," he said, laughing as he popped open his third beer.

Brian hung his head, chin resting on his dirty T-shirt. *It's the same old comment every night,* he thought. *If it's not that one, it's "Loosen your belt, Bri Bri, here comes another ten pounds," or "Why can't you be like your sister?" or "If you keep eating like that, I'll have to take out a bank loan just to put food on the table."*

Brian turned around and plopped himself down at the worn oval table where dinner was about to begin. He put three slices of pizza on the paper plate and grabbed a cola. Getting up from the table, he went to the living room and fell into the couch with his pizza and cola to watch television.

Brian sat in silence eating his meal as if there were no one else in the house. *Sometimes I get so tired of listening to my dad talk to me that way. I wish he weren't here. But I guess he works hard all day and when he comes home he's got to take it out on someone, so it might as well be me.*

Brian began to choke on his food. He had just shoveled half a slice of pizza into his mouth before he had even swallowed the first half. "Slow down," his father screamed from the kitchen. "Slow down before you choke to death." At that, Brian took one big painful gulp and sent his cheek-puffing mouthful of food down his throat.

"Are you okay, Brian?" his mother asked anxiously. "Are you okay? Don't eat so fast. Just take your time."

Madison murmured "pig" under her breath.

"I heard that," her mother said, snapping back at Madison. "You're not to speak about your brother that way!"

"Well," she snickered. "That's what he is. He's a pig! He eats like a pig and he looks like a pig. It makes me want to puke when I watch him eat." Brian just kept on eating, pretending not to be bothered by his sister's harsh words. Besides, he was used to it.

"That's enough," Charlotte screamed. She stood up and began throwing the paper plates into the trash. "Whose turn is it to clean up the kitchen?" she demanded. It seemed all she did was try to keep Brian and Madison from arguing.

"It's Brian's. It's Brian's," Madison yelped. "It's Brian's turn." No sooner had she said that than she got up and ran upstairs to her room, slamming the door behind her. Brian's dad shook his head.

"I don't know what's up with that girl lately. Have you noticed how she's been eating? She seems to just push the food around on her plate. When she takes a bite half of it comes back on the fork. I don't know who the heck she's trying to fool."

"I know, Marshall. What do you think we should do about it?" Charlotte glanced at Brian, who was all ears. "I'll talk about it with you later."

"Oh come on, you never let me hear the good stuff," he said, waiting to hear the rest of his parents' conversation.

"This is none of your business." Charlotte said. You shouldn't be listening to our conversation anyway."

"How can I help it? I'm right here in front of you."

"Cut the sarcasm. You just mind your manners," his father said, glaring at Brian.

Brian stood there stiff as a board. He knew if he said one more word his father would start yelling at him, and he hated the mean things he always said. *If I'm lucky he won't go on about it,* he thought hopefully.

His dad just stared at him for a moment and as soon as he was about to continue with Brian, Charlotte broke in to divert the potential disaster.

"Maybe she's just not feeling well." Marshall slowly looked toward Charlotte, directing his angry look at her instead of Brian.

Thanks, Mom, Brian said to himself.

"Well, I guess she's just going through one of those stages," Marshall said. "Thin is in, you know," he said shrugging his shoulders.

"Yes, I know, but she's lost so much weight lately. Maybe we should have a talk with her," Charlotte continued.

"Whatever you want to do, babe. She's your daughter," he said. He strolled out of the kitchen back to his favorite place in front of the TV and settled in for the evening.

"Give your mother a hand with the kitchen," he yelled at Brian. "You do a better job than Madison does anyway."

At least there's something I can do well. Brian stood up and began helping his mother with the trash. There were two slices of pizza to save.

"Put the leftover pizza in the fridge. I am going to sit and relax my back," his mother said getting a cigarette from the pack.

"Okay," Brian replied.

Brian began to put the leftover slices into a plastic food storage bag, when he thought, *"waste not, want not," that's what Mom always says.* And he proceeded to eat the last two slices of pizza. He never felt like he had had enough to eat unless he felt stuffed.

"All done, son?" she asked as she got up from her chair.

"You bet, Mom," he mumbled, as a bit of pizza sauce dribbled from his lower lip.

"You're such a good son. I don't know what I'd do without you. What more could a mother ask for?"

"Can I have an extra piece of cake for helping with the kitchen two nights in a row? Can I? Please!" His mother could never resist Brian when he pleaded for extra food. His chubby cheeks looked so cute to her. *Like an angel,* she thought.

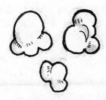

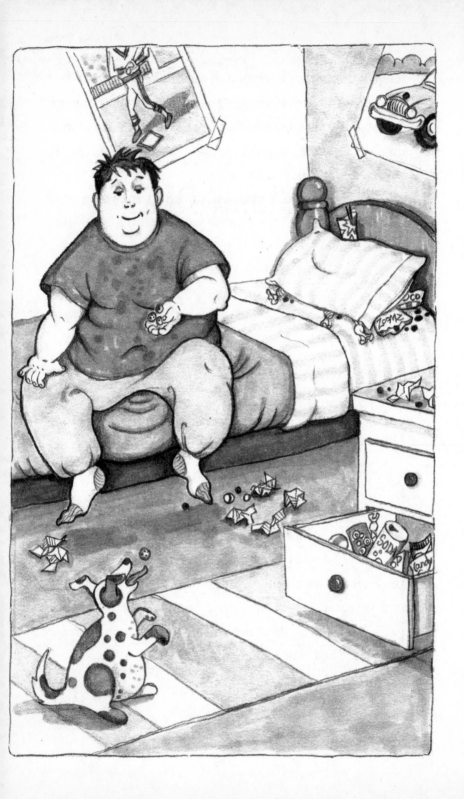

The Stash Drawer

Brian sat on the edge of his too-narrow bed, which creaked in protest. He noticed that his feet dangled an inch from the floor. *Pretty soon I'm going to be able to sit on the bed and touch both feet to the floor at the same time,* he thought as he dipped his toes to the floor. *Strange how my legs grow . . . I wonder if they would grow faster if I ate more. I bet I'll be seven feet tall before I'm thirteen. I better watch it or I'll be so tall people won't like me.*

I think people don't like other people when they're real different, he thought. *Most of the people I go to school with all look about the same. Some have brown hair, some have black hair, and some have blond hair, but they all kind of look alike. The other kids tease or are just plain mean to the ones who are real different. I don't like being*

teased or treated differently, he thought. *I just want to be
like the other kids.*

*Sometimes when I'm with Josh, the other kids make
fun of us because Josh is shorter than everybody in our
class and I'm fatter. I get so tired of that. Sometimes it
makes me feel . . .* Suddenly, there was a knock at the door.
Brian looked up and the door flung open. Madison stood
at the doorway with her blue and white cheerleading
outfit on and an angry look on her face.

"Hey," she snapped at Brian. "Have you seen my Jack
Jet CD? I was listening to it yesterday and now it's not
there. I always leave it in the same place in my room
sitting right on my nightstand. I need it for cheerleading.
Did you take it?"

"Can't you wait until I say 'come in'? You didn't even
give me a chance to say 'come in.' You're always walking
in on me. You better stop doing that or I'm going to tell."

"So what," she said defiantly. "Who cares? No one will
do anything anyway. No one cares what I do. Well, have
you seen my CD or not?" she screeched.

Brian heaved his body forward and with a smirking
grin snapped, "No, I haven't seen your stupid Jack Jet CD,
and if I had, I wouldn't tell you anyway. After what you
said to me at dinner tonight do you think I'd help you?"

"Come on, Brian, I was just kidding," she moaned. "I
didn't mean anything by it."

"Kidding!" he groaned. "It's not very funny. Did you see me laughing?"

"Okay!" Madison replied with a snap. "Okay. Are you sure you haven't seen my CD?"

"No, I told you. No!"

"Well then, will you help me look for it? I need it for tonight."

"Can't you see I'm busy? I've got things to do." Madison looked at him sitting on the corner of the bed looking like a big bump on a small log.

"Forget it. Just forget it!" she wailed. "I'll find it myself." She slammed the door behind her as she stamped out of the room.

A second later Madison suddenly opened the door, stuck her head in, and said, "By the way, I take it back. I'm going to call you whatever I want, Fatso!" This time she slammed the door twice as hard.

Brian slumped back over the bed and ended up on his back with his eyes staring straight up at the light fixture that hung over his bed. "Man, I hate her. I really do. I wish she was dead. Maybe she's not really my sister," he mumbled aloud. "Maybe her real parents will come and pick her up someday and I can live in peace."

Rumps was sitting in the corner listening to all the sounds that were going on. Rumps suddenly barked at Brian when Brian started talking to himself.

"Shhh," Brian said. "Be quiet before Dad starts pounding on the ceiling. You know he gets mad at me every time you start barking. He said if you do that one more time I have to get rid of you. Do you want that to happen? Do you?"

Rumps lifted his ears, cocked his head, and stared at Brian as if he really knew what Brian was talking about. Rumps stopped barking.

Brian had found Rumps a couple of blocks from his house in a dirty alley. He was a scrawny mutt with fleas, matted hair, and a hurt front paw. Brian could see parts of his brown and white fur were torn out, probably from dog fights. Brian often heard the dog fights that took place in the middle of the night. But he didn't care how Rumps looked or how he got that way. The dog liked Brian and Brian liked him. Brian was determined to keep this dog.

Brian brought him home the same day he found him and begged his father and mother to let him keep the dog. His father had told him absolutely not, but after twenty minutes of pleas and moaning and groaning, he won out, with his dad having begrudgingly lost the battle to a persistent son and a nagging wife.

"But if that dog makes a mess or gets in my way, he goes, and that's final." Marshall said, waving them away and stomping out of the room.

"What are you going to call him, Brian?" his mother asked gently.

"I don't know. Maybe I should name him after Dad since he let me keep him."

"Perfect. You can call him 'grumpy.'" They both laughed. "Or 'grumps' for short."

"I know," Brian said with excitement, "I'll call him 'Rumps.' It sounds like 'grumps.'"

"And every time I hear the name, I'll think of your father," Brian's mom said with a smile.

Brian proceeded from that moment forward to take care of Rumps. He took the thorn out of his paw, gave him a bath, dried him off, and brushed out his hair. He fed Rumps five times a day, just as often as Brian ate himself.

"Come on Rumps," he'd yell. "It's feedin' time." Rumps would come running, crashing into his bowl, sending his food everywhere. In time, Rumps got the hang of it and made his way to the bowl without knocking everything over.

Rumps had never had it so good. He ate every bit of the food that was given to him. As the weeks went by Rumps learned to run to his bowl every time Brian came into the house. As the months went by Rumps no longer dashed to the bowl, but rather waddled to the bowl as any plump dog would. And if it's true that a dog looks like its owner, then clearly Rumps had been put on this earth to be with Brian, his friend and master.

"Come here," Brian called as he clapped his hands at Rumps. "I've got a treat for you." Brian rolled over on the bed and reached into his nightstand and out of it came, as if it were magic, a bag of candy-coated peanuts. Rumps sat at the foot of the bed panting, ears high, tail wagging, and tongue hanging. He had seen these treats before—many times before. As a matter of fact, Brian and Rumps shared something to eat every night. All Rumps had to do was lift himself up just a little bit on his hind legs, stick his tongue out, and the treat was his. Though it was difficult at Rumps's size to do such a strenuous trick, he did so every night. Night after night, for his best friend, Brian.

Brian lay on the bed, stomach down, as he hurled the candies one-by-one into Rumps's gaping mouth. With each toss Rumps received the treats with great enthusiasm, knowing that there was more for the begging.

"Good boy," Brian praised. "Good boy. Here, want another one? Whoops, go get it! It's over there in the corner." Rumps scampered to retrieve the sloppily thrown treasure that awaited him on the floor in the corner of the room. "Good dog," Brian mumbled, having gobbled a handful while Rumps was getting his treat. And with two final tosses, one into Rumps's mouth and one into Brian's, the game was over.

"Here. See, Rumps," said Brian, his palms extended in front of him so that Rumps could see them. "All gone." Rumps cocked his head one more time and with ears raised higher than ever before, gave Brian his famous "what's going on?" look. If Rumps could have talked, Brian would have heard him say, "Just open your magic drawer, Brian. I know there's more in there. Come on, let's not stop now, I'm having too much fun." As if Brian knew what Rumps was thinking, he said aloud, "No more tonight, Rumps. There'll be more tomorrow."

You can't let dogs have too much candy, Brian said to himself. *All that stuff's not good for him.* Brian stood up with the empty candy bag still in his hand.

"Well, Rumps, where should I hide the candy bag? We don't want anybody to find out what's going on up here with our stash drawer of candy treats. If they find the empty bag they'll know for sure .... Let's see," he said with a puzzled look on his face. A moment later he exclaimed, "I know, I'll put it inside my school book. No one will find it there. On my way to school, I'll just throw it away. What do you think of that, Rumps?"

Rumps gave him an approving look as Brian walked over to his books. He flattened out the candy bag, opened his English book, and placed the bag neatly between the pages.

"There, Rumps," Brian giggled aloud, "no one will ever know it's ..." At that moment there was a knock on the door.

"Brian, can I come in?"

"Just a second, Mom." Brian slammed the book tightly over the candy wrapper. Brian hid his candy wrappers all over his room so his mother wouldn't find them. Rumps skidded his way over the hardwood floor and went crashing into the door where the sound of the knock had come from. Recovering from his tumble immediately, Rumps sat panting and waited for the arrival of the visitor.

"Come on in, Mom. Sorry, I was just finishing getting dressed."

Brian had already put on his favorite oversized T-shirt and sweatpants when he had first walked in his room. But he couldn't tell his mom what he was *really* doing. *It's not much of a lie*, he thought to himself. *She doesn't* really *care anyway.*

Brian's mom walked in and sat at his desk in the only chair in the room. It made a groaning, creaking noise as she settled into the chair.

"Well, Brian, tomorrow is Saturday and let's make it your day. Let's celebrate your report card. So what would you like to do? The usual?"

"YEAH," Brian exclaimed. "Yeah!"

"First, we'll go have some breakfast with all your favorites—biscuits, sausage, and pancakes with lots of syrup. And then we'll go play miniature golf."

Brian loved to play miniature golf. He didn't have to move very fast. He never got a chance to play football, basketball, or baseball because he spent most of his time sitting on the bench.

"Maybe we can go to that new restaurant on the other side of the hill. You know the one with the big kettle pot in front. I believe it's called The Brass Kettle. What do you think about that?"

"Is it any good? Do they serve a lot of food?" Brian asked.

"Brian," his mother said with a tone of exasperation. "Just because a restaurant serves a lot of food doesn't mean that it's good."

"Well, I'd rather go to Herb's Hamburgers anyway. They've got those giant double-thick hamburgers with cheese. Plus I'm dying for a chocolate shake. I've been thinking about their chocolate shakes all week long." Brian's mother laughed aloud.

"Well, it's your day, and you can have whatever you want."

"Thanks, Mom. Thanks a lot."

"Come on, get in bed. It's getting late." Brian climbed into bed. He rolled onto his squeaking bed and settled in for the night.

"Sleep tight and don't let the bed bugs bite," his mom said as she waddled down the hall. Brian could hear her heavy footsteps as she lumbered down the stairs.

"Good night, Mom," he called after her.

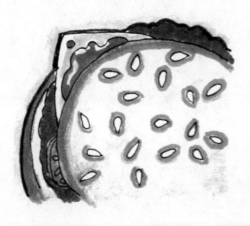

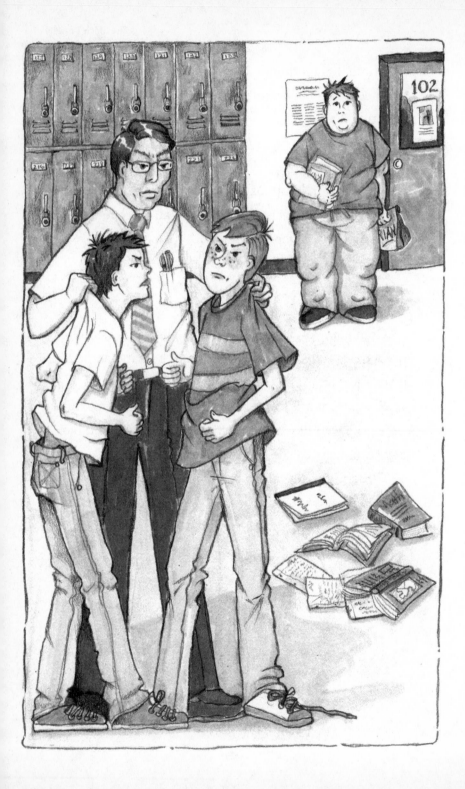

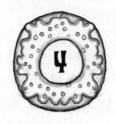

Trouble

Just as his mother promised, Brian had his special day on Saturday. His father didn't go with them as he'd said he would. He had a real bad headache and said that he needed to spend the day relaxing on the couch. Madison was nowhere to be found, but that didn't bother Brian. It wasn't her grades that earned the special day, so why should she have the fun that goes along with it?

In spite of his father's absence, Brian still had a great time. He was accustomed to spending most of his time with his mom anyway. They were pals and there was no taking that away from him.

Brian spent the next day playing with Rumps, doing his homework, watching TV, playing video games, and eating and eating and eating. Since there was nothing else to do except go to the park and watch the other kids play, he'd rather stay with Rumps and his stash drawer.

When the alarm went off Monday morning Brian lumbered out of bed, both bare feet smacking the floor at the same time. He went through his usual routine of getting ready for school: he brushed his teeth, washed his face, combed his hair, and grabbed a before-breakfast snack out of his private stash drawer.

He also had gone through his usual routine of going to the closet door, opening it, and making his clothes selection for the day. Brian had lots of clothes to choose from: brown and black pants, jeans, red and blue shirts, and various shoes to match. But he always went to his trusty old sweatpants, oversized T-shirt, and sneakers. All the rest of his clothes just didn't fit him anymore.

Every once in a while he would grab one of his pairs of pants out of the closet and try putting them on just to see if they might fit. But after losing yet another tug-of-war with his clothes, he would have to struggle out of them and hang them back up, to be tried on again some other time. The sweatpants covered him up so no one could see the plumper parts so easily. At least that's what Brian thought. For the moment, his trusty T-shirt and sweatpants would serve him just fine.

"I don't care how I look," he would say, not really meaning it. *I could wear those clothes if I wanted to, but they're just a little bit too tight. I'll lose weight and will fit into them someday.*

With that thought, Brian would grab his books, gobble down his breakfast, and head for school. Brian usually had donuts or sugar-frosted-something for breakfast. He liked having a diet soda in the morning. He felt like it gave him energy for the rest of the day.

Brian sat on the bus that took him on a seventeen block ride to Overton Junior High School. He sat at the window, not speaking with anyone, looking at all the cars that passed by and watching the other kids who either rode their bikes or skateboards or just walked to school.

Suddenly he flung open the window and yelled, "Josh, hey Josh!" But Josh, who was riding his bike, didn't hear him.

Josh was Brian's only friend at school. Sometimes Brian would go over to Josh's house after school and hang out. Once he even stayed overnight at Josh's house. He put the bus window back up and went back to his sightseeing. As usual, right around halfway to school Brian would open up his lunch to see what his mom had packed him. Today she packed two store-bought turkey sandwiches, potato chips, half-a-dozen cookies, some marshmallow-filled pies, and a chocolate candy bar. After surveying what was for lunch, he would close the bag back up and intend not to open it again until lunchtime. But after a minute or so Brian would, as usual, open the bag, reach in and grab a pre-school snack. This morning's chocolate candy bar would do just fine.

"Okay, everybody!" the bus driver yelled. "No pushing or shoving. Everyone have a great day."

So, pushing and shoving, everybody made their way off the bus. Brian always waited for everyone to get off the bus before he even stood up. He grabbed all of his books and his lunch and walked toward the front. "Hey, Brian," Mr. Roberts said. "How's my favorite student today?"

"Fine, Mr. Roberts. How are you doing?"

"I'm great. I'm having a wonderful day. Say, you know summer is a ways off, but do you have any thoughts or plans on what you want to do?"

"Oh, the usual," Brian replied with a sigh in his voice.

"Summer school again," Mr. Roberts exclaimed. "Don't you ever get tired of that?"

"Nah, there's nothin' else to do anyway."

"Well, what about summer camp or the local boys club. I'm sure you must have some friends to spend time with over the summer. Couldn't you do something like that?"

"That's kids stuff. It's stupid. Plus, my friend Josh always goes to stay with his grandma in Chicago."

Mr. Roberts reached over, patted Brian's shoulder, and said good-bye. Brian jumped to the sidewalk from the bus, making a loud thud. At that moment, Josh raced up on his bike coming to a screeching halt six inches away from Brian.

"Hey, look out! You could have killed me."

"No way!" Josh said with a voice of pure confidence. "This baby's got double lock brakes. I could have stopped closer, but I didn't want you throwing your books up all over my Mean Machine."

"Mean Machine? Is that its name?"

"Yeah, I decided I'm gonna be a professional motorcycle rider when I grow up. If you're gonna own a motorcycle, you've gotta give it a name. So I thought I'd start with my bicycle. What do you think?"

"Of course," Brian said sarcastically. "Last week you were going to be an astronaut and the week before a marine biologist. What next?"

"I don't know. Who cares," Josh mumbled. "What difference does it make? I'm never going to get out of this dumb old school anyway. By the way, can I borrow your math homework? I ... um ... uh ... um ..., well, I lost it on the way to school and I need to turn it in today. You know Mr. Paterson said that if I miss turning in my homework one more time I'll have to go talk to the principal."

"Josh, why don't you do your homework?"

Josh looked away from Brian as soon as the words came out of Brian's mouth. Josh had been having problems in school the last two years. He used to really like school. Then suddenly, for what seemed like no reason to Josh, his mom and dad started fighting a lot. Even though he would stay in his room and try to do his homework, he couldn't concentrate. In a short time, Josh went from all "A"s and "B"s to "D"s and "F"s. He just didn't seem to care anymore. He'd gaze out the window when he was sitting in class and didn't even listen to what the teachers were saying.

When he got home from school he had to help around the house. His mom said he had to help now that he was the man of the house. He really didn't want to be the man of the house, but when his mom and dad separated and were later divorced, it was just him and his mother. Somebody had to be in charge.

Josh missed his dad a lot. He hadn't heard from him ever since he left. For months after his dad left, Josh would go home and ask his mom if Dad was coming home. She would ignore him as if he weren't there. It seemed like all she did these days was sit around the house and watch television. If he did something that bothered his mother she would go into a rage.

"You're just like your father. Good for nothing. I don't even know why I had a kid. Men are just no good."

After a while Josh began to believe his mother. He was good for nothing.

"Josh, hey, Josh. Are you deaf? I've been talking to you. You haven't heard one darn word I said."

"I'm sorry, Brian. I was thinking about my dad."

"Have you heard from him?"

"Nope."

"Think you will?"

"I don't know. Mom says he's no good. She says he's never comin' back." He looked at Brian.

"Come on, Brian, what about that homework. Can I borrow it? What do you say?"

"Sure, Josh," Brian said sympathetically. "What are friends for?"

Brian handed his homework over to Josh and began walking toward the entrance of Overton Junior High. He knew it was wrong, but his friend needed help, so why not.

Overton Junior High School's buildings were all made of reddish brown brick, and the entrance had a big clock tower in it. To get inside the school Brian and Josh walked through the clock tower and under an archway to where the rest of the kids were all heading for their classes.

Josh parked his bike and carefully locked it where all the rest of the kids left their bikes. A year before, Josh had forgotten to lock his bike, and when he came out after school it was gone. His mom had been furious with him.

"My goodness Josh, what a stupid thing for you to do. We haven't got the money to buy you another bike with that father of yours not sending us any money, and I can't be bothered driving you back and forth to school. What are we going to do now?"

Fortunately, Josh's grandparents had heard about what had happened and sent him money for a new bike.

"Hey, Josh," Brian yelled as Josh was just finishing locking up his bike. "You want to do something after school?"

"I can't. I've got band practice."

"Oh yeah, I forgot," Brian moaned. "When are you going to give that up? One of these days that tuba is going to crush you to death." Josh was only five feet tall and as skinny as a rail. "I don't even know how you can make a sound out of that thing. There isn't enough air in you to blow out a candle, let alone a tuba. I think you ought to be a piccolo player instead. In fact, you look like a piccolo."

"Oh yeah, well you ought to be a tuba player. You look like a tuba!"

They both laughed and began walking their separate ways to class.

"See you later, Josh."

"See ya, Brian."

As Josh was saying good-bye to Brian, he turned his head and bam . . . ran right into Kyle, one of his least favorite people at Overton Junior High.

"Watch it, you stupid idiot," Kyle snapped, pushing Josh across the hall. "Where do you think you're going?"

Brian froze in his tracks, stood and stared at both of them, afraid of what was about to happen.

Josh took the books that he was holding and hurled them across the hall into Kyle's face.

"I'm going to kill you, you jerk!" Josh screamed. And at that, he ran and jumped on Kyle, causing them both to tumble to the floor. They both rolled back and forth in the hallway yelling and screaming at each other.

"I'm gonna kill you," Josh bellowed again.

"You asked for it," Kyle yelled.

It didn't take more than a few seconds for a crowd to gather around them. Each member of the crowd picked the one that they wanted to win and cheered him on.

"Get 'um, Kyle," yelled one of them.

"Come on, Josh. Knock 'um out," yelled another.

"Put your knee in his stomach, Josh."

As everybody in the crowd was yelling for one or the other, suddenly, as if it came from nowhere, both Josh and Kyle felt the grip of a hand on each of their necks. In one motion they were suddenly pulled apart.

"All right, that's enough from the both of you," said the principal.

"He pushed me first," returned Kyle.

"Did not," snapped Josh.

They both began their arguing all over again as they tried to take punches at one another. But it was useless as the firm grip of the principal remained on the back of each of their necks.

"I want everybody to go to their classes. Let's break it up."

Moans and groans sounded as the crowd of students went their separate ways.

"He could have busted him up real good," said one of them.

"Oh, yeah! Kyle would have killed him."

"No way, man. I've seen Josh fight. That guy's mean."

"I don't know what this is all about, but I want both of you in my office right now," the principal repeated firmly.

"But . . ."

"Right now!" barked the principal.

Brian never moved, even when the crowd blocked his view. He stood and watched as the principal marched both of them away.

"Darn that Josh," Brian mumbled to himself. "If he keeps fighting like that he's gonna get expelled, and then who will I hang out with?" Brian turned around and walked toward his class shaking his head. *Darn that Josh.*

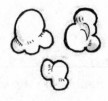

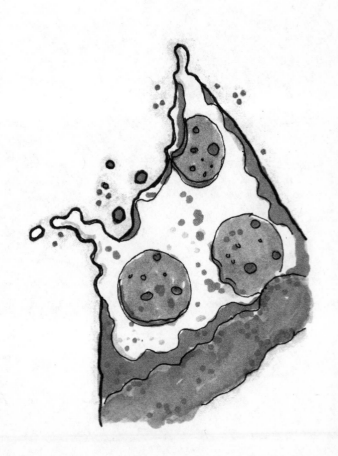

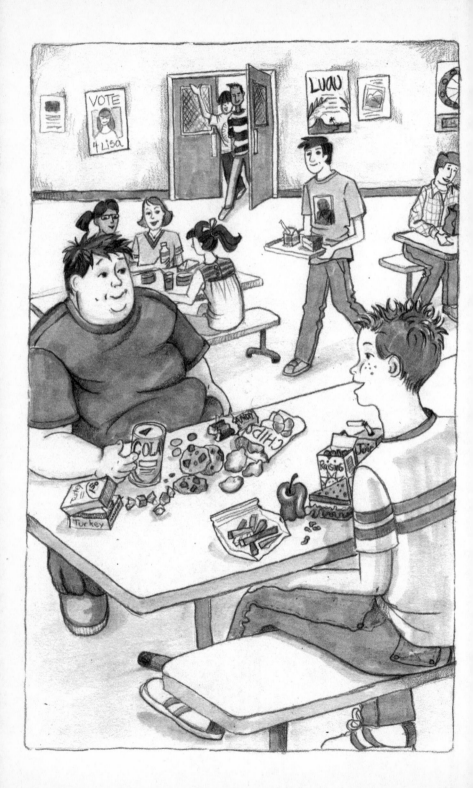

There's a New
Kid in Town

Even though the first day of summer vacation
was two weeks away, the early morning sun shined with
enough warmth to suggest summer's early arrival.

Brian walked down the hallway, which was
illuminated by the sun's bright light. He always marveled
at how the light beams made strange shapes on the walls
around him. As he walked along the hallway, his body
blocked the illuminations that crept through the glass
that arched over the hallway. With each step Brian made,
a different-shaped reflection appeared. He stooped down
or stretched on his toes to make the shapes even weirder
than they already were. Sometimes the shapes looked
like monsters from movies that he had seen. Other times

they looked like giant blobs rolling down the walls. As he walked, he laughed at himself and what he was doing.

Brian stopped in the middle of the glass-covered hallway and began moving slowly, waving his arms to make funny shapes on the wall. He suddenly lowered his arms, remembering how he used to make Josh laugh when he made his funny shapes.

It had been about two months since Brian had seen Josh. Ever since the time the principal caught Josh fighting in the hall with Kyle things had only gotten worse. After that fight, Josh had detention for a whole week, and not more than two weeks had passed before Josh picked another fight in the boy's bathroom.

"You gotta stop fightin' with everybody," Brian pleaded. "If you keep this up, you're gonna get kicked out of school."

"So what, I don't care. They're nothing but jerks going to this school anyway," Josh replied. Brian frowned. "Except for you, Brian. You're okay. You're a good guy."

"If you get kicked out of school, you'll have to go to summer school to make it up."

"No way, man. I'll run away first."

Just as if Josh wanted that to happen, three months later he got kicked out of school for starting a fire in one of the trash cans. When Brian tried to call Josh at his home, his mom answered the phone. She told him that Josh had run away and that the police were looking for him. She said something about sending him away when they caught him.

Brian had not seen or heard from Josh since the day before he'd started the fire. He called Josh's house again, but this time the phone was disconnected. He missed Josh a lot. Brian didn't talk to anyone about it, he just missed him. He missed his only friend at school.

Leaving the hallway, Brian walked around the corner, entered the door marked C-3, and took his usual seat in Ms. Diaz's class. Just as he sat down the bell rang.

"Class," the chairs and desks continued to make noise as Ms. Diaz waited for the classroom to become silent. "Before we start with today's assignments, I have a surprise for you. In spite of the fact that the school year is about to end, we have a new student. His name is Jeffrey Armstrong and he's just moved here with his family from a city in Arizona called Phoenix." The whole class turned around and stared at the new face sitting at the back of the classroom.

"Since there are only two weeks of school left, Jeffrey's not going to have much of a chance to get to know all of you before school lets out. So, I'd like all of you to make an effort to get to know him. Summer can be very lonely without friends. Will someone volunteer to show Jeffrey around for the next couple of days? Raise your hands."

Ms. Diaz stared at the class as they sat motionless. By this time all the students had a set routine between classes and after school. They couldn't be bothered with the job of showing some new kid around.

"Okay," she said. "I'll pick somebody. Brian."

"But..."

"Thank you, Brian. Now, let's get started on our assignment."

At lunchtime, during the forty-five minutes during which the students were supposed to eat, Brian sat in his usual place, where he always ate what was left of his lunch, formerly with Josh, but today Brian had a job to do. Just as he began to take the first bite out of his sandwich, Jeffrey walked up.

"Hi! Well, Brian, I found you, no problem."

Brian had told Jeffrey where to meet him for lunch after he left Ms. Diaz's class. Brian didn't look up. He bit down on his sandwich, started to chew, and then took a gazing look at Jeffrey, who stood before him.

"Sit down, Jeffrey."

"Thanks, Brian. Just call me Jeff."

"Okay, whatever."

"Thanks for taking the time to show me around."

"I was going to volunteer, but Ms. Diaz called on me just before I was going to raise my hand. So why did your folks decide to move out here, anyway?"

"Well, my dad is an engineer and he got a promotion. Mom wasn't real happy about it, though. She didn't want me and my two sisters to change schools this late in the year."

"Two sisters," groaned Brian. "Two sisters. I can barely handle the one I've got. I would have run away from home years ago if I had two sisters!"

"Aw, they're not so bad. We fight every once in a while, but sometimes they're my best friends. Dawn is a year younger than me and Samantha is four years older. She's going to graduate from high school next year. She wants to be a doctor."

"How old are you?" Brian asked.

"I just turned thirteen."

"I'm twelve-and-a-half. We're almost the same age. What have you got for lunch?" Brian asked with anticipation.

Jeff opened his lunch bag and placed everything on the table where they were sitting. "I've got a tuna sandwich, some carrot sticks, a box of raisins, and an apple."

"That's all?" belted Brian in a loud voice. "That's it? What are they trying to do, starve you to death?"

Jeff leaned his head to the side with a puzzled look on his face. He didn't understand what Brian meant. He thought he had a great lunch.

"What's for dessert?"

"My apple is my dessert," he said. "I always have a piece of fruit for dessert."

"Oh boy," Brian said sarcastically. "What a drag you are. My friend Josh always had good stuff for dessert. He never ate it so he always gave it to me."

"Well, I like my dessert," Jeff replied enthusiastically, "and I'm going to keep it."

Brian let out a huff and a sigh and finished eating his lunch of chips, pre-made, store-bought sandwiches, chocolate-chip cookies, and of course the candy he always kept with him. His lunch always took up all of the space in his backpack, unless his mom gave him money to buy lunch at school. Brian liked the sack lunch because he got more food. "Let's get started, Jeff. Lunchtime's almost over and Ms. Diaz said to show you around the school."

"Great. Where to first, Brian?"

"To get an ice cream, where else?"

Fifteen minutes later Brian had shown Jeff where the school library was, where the PE building was, and then returned with him to the most important building at the school, the lunchroom. The two boys seemed to be getting along great when Jeff said, "By the way, my mom said if I met anybody at school who I liked, I could invite them over for dinner on Saturday. How 'bout it? Would you like to come?"

"Who, me?" Brian asked with a startled voice. "You only invite friends over for dinner."

"Well, you are my friend. My newest friend."

Brian didn't know what to say. He didn't have many friends, and those he did have were just his friends at school. He never saw them outside of school and had never been invited to anyone's house for dinner, or for anything else for that matter, with the exception of Josh. After a moment, he said, "That would be great! I'll be there."

Wow, Brian thought, *dinner at a friend's house. A new friend.*

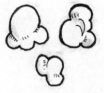

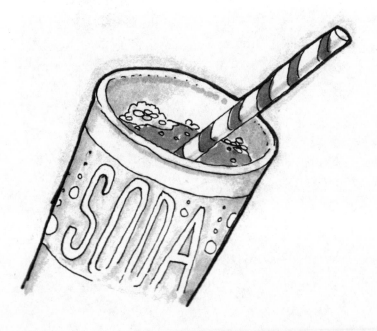

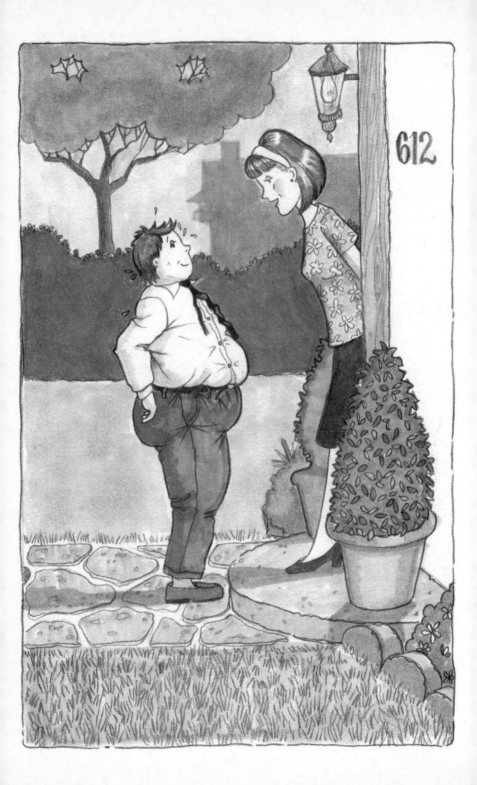

IF It's Not One Thing, It's Another

It was seven o'clock by the time Brian walked through the gate that led to the front door at 612 Croft Street. He was supposed to have arrived at six thirty for dinner at Mr. and Mrs. Armstrong's house. Jeff, his new friend from school, asked him to be a little early so that his family could meet him before they sat down to dinner. But as it turned out, Brian would be knocking on the door at the same time dinner was to be served.

The night was unusually hot and Brian was more than uncomfortable in his white shirt, tie, and black pants. He wanted to look especially nice so he could impress Jeff's family. But his shirt was sopping wet from perspiration, not only from the hot night, but from his anxiety at being late.

It wasn't totally his fault that he was late. There were just a few things that didn't go right. Brian had gone to his closet to pick out what he was going to wear. He reached in and got his best black pants, blue shirt, and favorite red and blue tie. He had just gotten the tie six months ago for his birthday and had only worn it once. Brian slipped on his black pants in the only way he could. He would sit on the edge of his bed, put both feet in his pants at the same time and with one mighty pull and many muffled grunts, he would bounce up and down as his pants rose to his hips. This was only the beginning of his frustrations.

Before his pants reached his waist he heard the sound of a long, loud rip. The seam on the inside of his right leg had split wide open. Whenever this happened, and it had happened before, a lot, he called it a "blowout."

"Oh no!" Brian yelled, with a loud tone of disgust in his voice. "Another blowout. That's the second pair of pants this week." *Could these pants have shrunk, too,* Brian thought.

He jumped down from the bed, pulled his pants down past his thick thighs, and stepped out of them as he walked across the floor to the closet in a marching step. Just as he reached the closet door the pants released their final grip on his foot and he angrily kicked them into the corner.

He looked in his closet for his last pair of black pants. *I'd better be careful with these,* he thought. *If I blow these out there'll be nothing nice to wear to dinner.*

Brian went back to his position at the edge of the bed, and with an attitude of determination he slowly pulled his pants up. As he did he lay back on the bed and, wiggle by wiggle, brought them safely around his waist.

Finally, he inhaled all the breath that he could, quickly snapped the pants, buckled the belt and gasped for air. Looking down, his stomach hid his belt buckle from view, but the tightness around his waist told him the task was complete.

He put his blue shirt on and began to button it as he stared in the mirror. "Darn it!" he yelled, noticing a big spot of spaghetti sauce on his shirt. "What a slob." *I can't go like this,* he thought to himself critically. *Why didn't Mom wash it? Now I can't wear it tonight.*

Brian ripped at the buttons, trying to take the shirt off, popping one of them off in the process. With one continuous motion, he pulled at his shirt and tossed it in the opposite corner from the one into which he had kicked the pants.

With time running out he hurriedly grabbed his only white shirt out of the closet, rammed his arms into the sleeves, and buttoned it to his neck. Brian heaved his shirt tails down the front of his pants and put the already knotted tie over his head and around his shirt collar.

At six thirty he went running down the stairs, his shirt trailing behind him, to get his dad, who had promised to drive him to Jeff's house.

"Dad, Dad, hey Dad, wake up, it's time to go. I'm going to be late." His dad didn't budge an inch from the couch where he had been lying all day. He just lay there as if he had no life in him. Brian leaned over the worn gray sofa and shook his dad's limp shoulders. "Dad, Dad, come on Dad, you promised. You promised to take me over to Jeff's house tonight."

"What . . . what . . . huh?" Brian's dad moaned. "What's going on? What's the trouble?"

"Dad, don't you remember? I'm having dinner tonight at Jeff's, my new friend. Please, Dad, come on, you promised," he pleaded.

Brian had told his mother and father of his newfound friend. He explained where Jeff and his family had moved from and how his mother underfed Jeff when she packed his lunches. His father had snorted at Brian's comment.

"Give me his phone number," he said sarcastically. "I'd like to call his mother and see if she wouldn't mind giving 'Toots' here a few lessons." He cocked his head toward Brian's mother. "She packs enough in your lunch to feed a small regiment." Charlotte just ignored his comment and sauntered away.

"Anyway, Dad, Jeff invited me over for dinner on Saturday. Will you take me?"

"You bet, Bri Bri. You've got my word on it."

Brian's father had promised him on more than one occasion to take him somewhere and never followed through. Those afternoon drinks just made him too tired.

But tonight his father lifted himself up on one elbow, raked his reddish hair back over his forehead, and let out a long moan.

"Oh, yeah, Brian, right, uh ..., why don't you get me my keys from the bedroom and bring me some aspirin from the medicine chest?"

"Right, Dad. Jeff's house is two miles past the school and our house is two miles before the school so that's four miles," he said lumbering up the stairs to his father's room. "It's already six thirty, so can we please hurry? I'm gonna be late." There was no reply.

Brian ran into the bedroom, grabbed the keys from his parents' night table, and rushed into the bathroom. Clutching the aspirin, he began to run downstairs. Just as he hit the foot of the stairs he tripped and fell. Brian made a loud thud as he hit the floor, groaning at the same time.

Slowly he got to his hands and knees and crawled a few feet, grabbed an armchair that was next to him, and pulled himself up. He was clutching the keys so tightly that he never let go of them, even when he fell. They left an indentation in his hand, which he noticed as he released them to give to his father.

"Okay, Dad, here they are. Let's go." Much to Brian's disappointment his father had fallen back asleep again. Any efforts to wake him were to no avail.

"Now what am I going to do?" moaned Brian loudly, hoping to wake his father. "I'll never get to Jeff's house."

At that moment Brian heard the front door open. He turned to see his mother and sister walking into the house.

"Hey, Mom!" Madison yelled. "There's an overstuffed penguin in the living room." She giggled at her own joke as she leaped up the stairs to her room, two steps at a time.

"Very funny," Brian yelled as Madison slammed her door.

"Mom, hurry. You gotta take me to Jeff's. I'm late. Dad promised to take me, remember? But I can't wake him up. Mom, please, please! You've got to hurry. I'm gonna be late."

Charlotte looked over to the couch where Marshall was sprawled. Sitting on the coffee table was an empty can of beer.

"Oh, Marshall, not again," she mumbled. "How could you? How could you?"

Brian pulled his mother outside the door as she was shaking her head in disgust.

"Okay, Brian," she snapped. "I'm coming. You won't be too late."

Charlotte wasn't the best driver and didn't know that side of town very well. It was a few minutes before seven when she finally pulled up to Jeff's house.

"Thanks, Mom," he said as he opened the car door and stepped onto the curb.

"You're welcome, Brian. Have a good time."

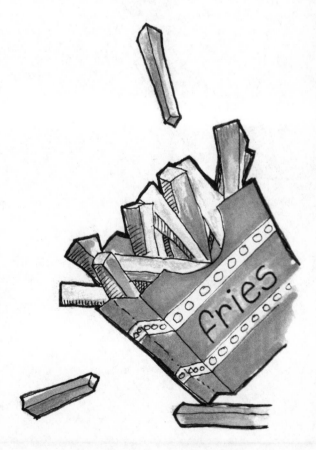

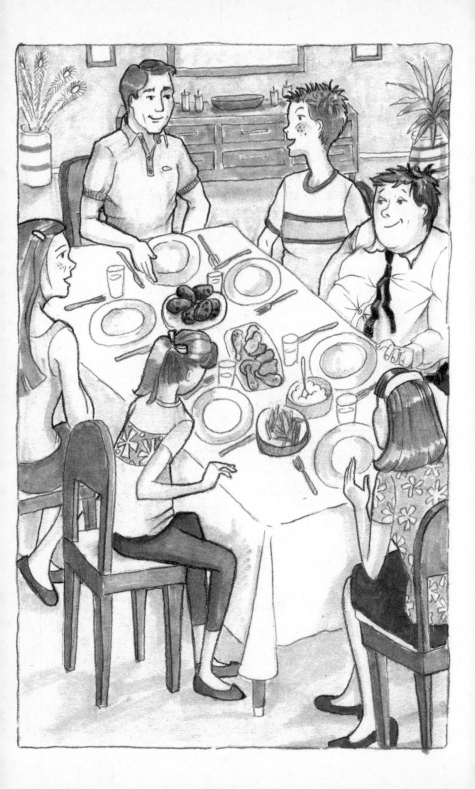

Meet the Armstrongs

Brian was about to knock on the door when he noticed his shirt was out of his pants again. He began stuffing his shirt back into his pants with his fat little hands. As he did, the door suddenly opened.

Before him stood a tall, attractively dressed woman. Brian stared up at her, with his hands still down the front of his pants, his mouth half open. With his bright red face matching the color of his tie, he sheepishly smiled at the woman in front of him.

"Hi," she said with a welcoming smile on her face. "Now I'll just bet that you're Brian," her right hand extended for a handshake. "I'm Mrs. Armstrong."

As soon as Brian stepped into the house, Jeff grabbed him and showed Brian around his new home. It wasn't a two-story house like Brian's. The whole house was on one level. Brian guessed that since they had just moved in they hadn't had a chance to unpack everything. There were still boxes in the half-painted hallways and bedrooms, all of them full of treasures that had been collected over the years. They had been moved across country and now needed to be unpacked and put away.

After Brian got over the embarrassment of his initial meeting with Mrs. Armstrong, he began to calm down and feel more comfortable. She didn't make a big deal over the incident at the door. Brian was grateful for that. He had felt bad enough over being late.

She showed him to a bathroom that was located next to the front door entrance in the hallway so he could tuck in his shirt, put some water on his hair, and straighten his tie. When he finished, he opened the bathroom door to find Jeff waiting for him.

"Hey, we were getting worried about you. What happened?"

"Uh, well, I, um, was doing my homework and I didn't realize how late it was." Brian didn't like telling the truth when something happened at home. His mom and dad got mad at him if he went around blabbing about things that went on. "I'm sorry I was late."

"Oh, that's okay. Do you want to see my room? It's right over . . ." Just then, Jeff's mother walked into the hallway from the dining room.

"Okay, boys, are you hungry? It's dinner time. Jeff, why don't you show Brian where to sit. I hope you kids are hungry."

Brian was starving. He followed Jeff to the beautifully set dinner table with its fresh flowers and white tablecloth. Just as he sat down in his seat, the rest of Jeff's family came into the room.

"Brian, these are my two sisters. This is my little sister, Dawn."

"I'm not little," she sneered back. "Hello. How are you doing?" she replied in a much calmer voice.

"And this is Samantha."

"Hello. Jeff's told me a lot about you."

"And this is my dad."

"Hello, Brian. You look nice. Do you always wear a tie to dinner?"

"Oh, sure, Mr. Armstrong. I wear one all the time."

Brian was glad that Mr. Armstrong noticed what he was wearing. He had only worn a tie one other time before, but that didn't matter, he was wearing a tie now.

Everyone began to sit around the table, Jeff's father at one end, his mother at the other, and his two sisters across from Jeff and Brian.

Brian was getting hungrier and hungrier. He hadn't had anything since his before-dinner snack at five o'clock. The chips and cookies were not going to hold him much longer.

Before him on the table sat a plate of chicken, some carrots, and baked potatoes. A bowl of apple sauce was directly in front of him. Brian wasn't a big fan of carrots or baked potatoes, but he liked chicken, especially if it was chicken nuggets. He didn't usually eat this kind of food. He was used to eating pizza, burgers, fries, and sweet stuff. Oh, how he liked sweet stuff. He was sure there was going to be more food than what was on the table. *Feeding a family of five plus a guest would certainly take more than this*, Brian thought to himself. He reached for the chicken just as Mrs. Armstrong said, "Well, since you're our guest, Brian, how about saying grace?" Brian jerked his hand back as a wave of nervousness ran through his body.

"Grace? I, um, uh . . . Sure, I guess." He looked around the table and saw all of their heads bowed down. A moment went by before Jeff lifted his head to see Brian straining to think of something to say.

"Hey, Mom," Jeff blurted. "Can I say grace?" The rest of the family had also felt Brian's awkwardness.

"Why don't you do that, Jeff. Brian, do you mind?"

"Ah . . . no, I don't mind."

"Jeff," his mother said after he finished saying grace, "Would you like to serve this evening?"

"Okay, Mom. Brian, why don't you pass me your plate?"

Jeff served Brian just as he served everyone at the table: two pieces of chicken, a scoop of carrots, and a baked potato. Brian stared at the plate before him. *Surely there must be more,* he thought. *This can't be all there is for dinner.*

But it became apparent to Brian that this was all there was for dinner. At that moment, Brian felt hunger in a way that he never had felt before. He knew he was still going to be hungry even after eating all that was on his plate. This made Brian feel empty and nervous.

"Would you like some bread?" Samantha asked, looking straight at Brian. *Bread,* he thought. *Bread and butter. Lots of bread and butter should take care of this empty feeling.* "Yes, thank you," he mumbled with his mouth full of chicken.

"We've got some warming in the oven. I'll get it." Samantha returned to the table with a covered basket and stood before him. "Here you go," she said. "My favorite kind of bread."

Brian peeled back the white cloth napkin to reveal, much to his dismay, wheat bread. *Plain old wheat bread,* he thought, *I hate wheat bread.* "Thanks," Brian replied. "My favorite." Grabbing one slice, he put it on his plate as his eyes began to search the table for some butter.

"Excuse me," Brian said. "May I have some butter?"

Dawn passed the butter to Brian. They all watched as he slathered his bread with about a half-inch thickness of butter. Brian liked butter and didn't think anything of using so much. Anyway, it covered the taste of the whole wheat brown bread.

As they sat around eating their dinner, each of them shared what had happened that day. In-between the sharing, one of them would ask a question of Brian: about the town, the surrounding area, and what kinds of things there were to do.

"Are there any good places to go swimming?" Dawn asked excitedly.

"Sure, there's the big pool at one of the parks and there are a couple of lakes at the other."

"Is there a place to go skateboarding around here?" Jeff blurted.

"Well, um, uh, yeah. I've only tried it a couple of times. But there's a big hill a few blocks from school where all the kids go skateboarding."

"Do you want to go to college when you graduate?" Samantha inquired.

"You bet. I'd like to be a lawyer. I watch television shows all the time about lawyers. The lawyer always gets them in the end. Plus, they make a bunch of money." Everyone at the table laughed.

"So, tell me, what does your father do?" questioned Mr. Armstrong.

"My dad works at the Ford plant. He's real important. Lots of men have to check in with him to get permission to do things. Sometimes they even call him at night and he has to go back to the plant. He works late a lot."

"Sounds real important," Mr. Armstrong replied.

"Well, I'm glad that Mr. Armstrong doesn't have to do that. We'd miss him if he got called away. Besides, we all like to have dinner together," Mrs. Armstrong said, with a concerned tone.

Everybody at the table kept asking Brian more questions about where to go shopping, where to go to the movies, and what kinds of things he liked to do. He liked all the attention he was getting. It made him feel good. It made him feel important.

As the evening passed, the whole family started telling him stories about what it was like in Arizona.

There was the time when Jeff and his dad went to the State Fair. Someone pulled the pin out of the chicken coop and all the girls were screaming as they tried to round up the chickens and put them back into their cages. They had both gone on the biggest roller coaster ride in Arizona and sat in the front seat.

"I was so scared," Jeff explained. "I thought I was going to . . ."

"Jeffrey!" his mother scolded him lovingly. Dawn covered her mouth as she giggled at what Jeff had started to say.

There was the trip the whole family had taken to the Grand Canyon, the Petrified Forest, and the Painted Desert. They had spent a week river rafting, hiking, camping, and horseback riding.

Jeff jumped up in the middle of his story about the trip to run and get something from his room. He came back with a rock clenched in his hand.

"See, Brian. This is called petrified wood. A long time ago it was a piece of a tree, but somehow it turned into rock."

There was last Christmas when they already knew that they were going to have to move to their new home. The Armstrongs threw a big family celebration. Relatives came from miles around, and the Christmas tree had lots and lots of presents under it.

Samantha, Dawn, and Jeff had put on a play for the family. When Jeff came out of the room with his Santa Claus outfit on, the pants were too long and he tripped, falling right on top of a big Christmas cake.

The family laughed along with Brian at the story of Jeff's clumsy fall.

"Okay," Mrs. Armstrong interjected. "Who's got kitchen duty tonight?"

"I doooo." Jeff moaned. He paused for a minute. "Hey, Samantha, can I trade days with you? I'll wash the dishes tomorrow if you wash for me tonight."

"Sure, Jeff, you've got a deal."

"Come on, Brian. Let's go to my room."

Jeff took Brian to his room. There were model airplanes, a collection of his favorite rocks, and posters of rock groups and skateboarders all over the walls. In

a corner, next to an unpacked box, stood a bunch
of trophies.

"What are those for?"

"Oh, I used to be in Little League."

"You mean you won all those?"

"All but one. The big one was for the first place team.
My dad coached that year, too. He's a great baseball
player. He taught me a lot."

"Your dad plays baseball, too?" Brian asked
with amazement.

"Yeah. He played baseball when he was in school and
his father taught him. He said as soon as we get settled
we'll try to find a league out here to play on."

Brian thought back. He could not remember a time
in his life when he and his father had even so much as
thrown a ball back and forth.

Dawn came running into the room.

"Hey, don't you know how to knock?" Jeff asked,
somewhat perturbed.

"Sorry, Jeff. You want me to go back out and knock?"

"No, that's all right. What's up?"

"You guys want to play a game? Mom and Dad said
they'd play. Samantha, too!"

"How 'bout it, Brian?" Jeff asked.

"Sure, what are we going to play?"

They all gathered around the dining room
table again.

"All right, everybody. How about an exciting game of Uno? I'll beat the pants off of you all," said Mr. Armstrong, with a grin on his face.

"What's Uno?" Brian asked. Dawn slapped her head with her open palm in response.

"Oh, you've got to be kidding."

"Dawn," Samantha said, giving her a loving push. "That's not nice."

It didn't take long for Brian to learn the game. The rest of the evening was full of friendly moans, groans, and kidding as the game went on. The more they played the game the more fun Brian had. For the first time in a long time, Brian had forgotten how hungry he had been.

"I think we had better wrap this up," Mrs. Armstrong said. "We need to get Brian home."

"Ah, Mom," Jeff whined. "Can't we play just one more game?"

Mrs. Armstrong glanced across the table at her husband. Brian saw the wink of his eye giving approval to the request.

"Okay, since you have a guest, one more game. Deal 'em! You're going to lose this one, sucker!" Mrs. Armstrong joked.

As predicted, she won. When the game was over, everyone helped clean up the table.

"How are you getting home, Brian?" Mr. Armstrong questioned. "Tell you what," he said not waiting for a reply. "Why don't Jeff and I drive you home. Since we're new in town it will give me a chance to see where you live and learn a little bit more about the city."

"Well, okay, sure."

"It was nice of you to come over for dinner," Mrs. Armstrong said. "Please come back again."

"This was great," Brian replied. "I will, anytime."

Mr. Armstrong piled Jeff and Brian into the car and with Brian giving directions headed for his house on the other side of town.

"Do you want us to wait until you get inside, Brian?" Mr. Armstrong asked.

"No, that's okay. Thanks for bringing me home, Mr. Armstrong."

"See you Monday, Brian."

"See you, Jeff. Thanks again. I had a really good time."

Brian walked to the front door very slowly. He hated that the evening was over tonight, and he hated what was waiting for him on the other side of the door.

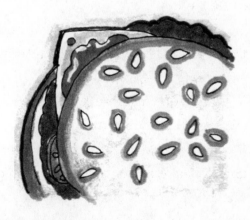

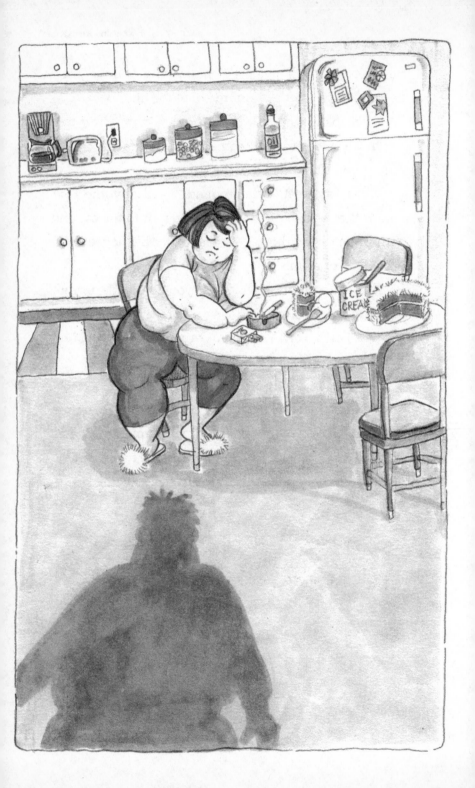

Yesterday and Today

It was 10:30 that evening before Brian got home. He walked into his dimly lit house to find a scene that he had viewed many times before. His father was still lying on the couch. He did not appear to have moved all evening. Brian would have thought that was the case, except for the many beer bottles sitting side by side with the others that had been there when he had left earlier that evening.

Brian began to walk toward the stairs when he noticed the light on in the kitchen. His feet fumbled as he changed direction and headed toward the light.

When he arrived he came upon another familiar sight. His mother was sitting at the kitchen table, an open gallon of fudge ripple ice cream in front of her. Beside the ice cream sat a platter that once held a whole, double-layered coconut cake that was now two-thirds gone. On a plate in front of her was a melting, half-eaten scoop of ice cream and the remnants of a piece of coconut cake.

Brian's mom sat with one elbow pressing into the walnut kitchen table, her forehead in the palm of her hand. Her thick, obese thighs hung over the edge of the chair. His mom's chunky feet were stuffed into a pair of badly worn pink house slippers and her other arm was extended, barely touching the ashtray that held a half dozen or so snuffed cigarette butts. One cigarette was smoldering freely at the edge of the ashtray. For as long as Brian could remember his mother had been big, but over the last few years she had become huge. He found the odor of the cigarettes, which she smoked constantly, to be unusually strong tonight.

"Hey, Mom. I'm home," he said, giving her a peck on the cheek.

"Hi, Brian," she answered nonchalantly, not even looking up.

"Mom, I had the best time at Jeff's house."

"That's nice."

"We ate dinner and we sat around and talked and we played a card game. Everyone in the family. And we . . ."

"I am so angry at your father. We haven't said three words all night. I'll tell you, Brian, I've had it with him. Just had it!"

"But, Mom, I was telling you about . . ."

"If it wasn't for you kids, I would have left that man a long time ago. Someone has got to take care of you kids, you know. He certainly can't do it. Who'd do it if I wasn't here? Sometimes I feel like leaving and never coming back. That's it. I just feel like chucking it all."

"But, Mom, I was telling you about tonight, over at Jeff's house."

"Oh, I know Brian. I'm sorry. I'm just fed up. And as if that wasn't enough, your lovely sister ran out of the house screaming about something. Heaven knows what it was. I've called all over; I can't find her anywhere. I'm going to strangle her when she comes home. *If* she comes home." She stopped for a moment and looked at Brian standing before her. "But you're my boy, Brian. You never cause me any problems and you're always here to keep me company. How about a piece of cake and some ice cream?"

Brian looked down at the remains on the table. He could have easily eaten it all. "No thanks, Mom, not tonight. I think I'm just going to go to bed." He made an about-face and left the kitchen.

"Don't wake Sleeping Beauty," she yelled with a sarcastic tone in her voice. "We wouldn't want to disturb your dad." Brian had already left the room.

"Come back, son," his mother cajoled. Brian stopped in his tracks and went back into the kitchen. His mother was smiling. "Sit down and keep me company for a little while. It's not a school night. Are you *sure* you won't have some ice cream and cake?"

Brian's stomach growled. He had almost forgotten about the measly dinner he had had at the Armstrongs. Suddenly, he felt hungry. "Okay," he said, sitting down.

"So the Armstrongs were nice, huh?" asked his mother, putting the remains of the cake on a paper plate in front of him. "Nice, how?"

"I dunno . . ." Brian mumbled, coconut cake muffling his words. "You know, nice . . . like, they play games, and they asked me a lot of questions about living here."

"They asked questions?" his mother asked. Her eyes got narrow, but that could just have been from the cigarette smoke.

"Yeah, questions," said Brian, too busy shoveling cake into his mouth to notice the anger in his mother's eyes. "And they asked me if I'd go back and have dinner there again sometime," he said, his eyes shining with anticipation.

"Well, we'll just see about that," his mom snapped. "We'll just have to see about your new friends, Mr. and Mrs. Nosy Armstrong and all the little Nosy Armstrongs, with all their nosy questions!"

"It wasn't like that Mom," Brian began, but his mother silenced him.

"You just remember to keep our family's business inside these four walls. Use that mouth for eating, that's what it's for, not for blabbing all our family secrets all over town."

Brian pushed his plate away. There was still some cake left, but he didn't feel like eating it anymore. He left the kitchen and began to climb the stairs, ignoring the rest of his mother's comments.

She always tells me to keep family secrets, Brian thought to himself. *Some* secrets. *Like Dad drinks too much and my sister's an exercise nut? Who the heck wants to tell people about that?* He entered his room, closing the door behind him and flopped himself face down on his bed.

Rumps dragged himself toward the edge of the bed and awaited the opening of the magical stash drawer. After a few moments Rumps lifted his paw and began scratching the bed, making a whining noise at the same time.

"Stop it, Rumps, not tonight." Rumps continued and with a flick of his wrist Brian leaned forward and pushed Rumps away.

The dog didn't understand, but sensed that something was wrong. In the entire time that Brian had been his owner he had never ignored Rumps or pushed him away.

Whimpering his way to the corner, Rumps let out a soft whine. He turned around and let out a huff from his nose and settled in for the night.

This was a strange night, thought Brian. Even though it was almost summer, a heavy rain had begun pounding on the roof shortly after he had arrived home. An occasional crackle of thunder separated the patter of raindrops as they struck the house. He rolled over on his bed and stared up at the ceiling. The evening at Jeff's reminded him of his family a long time ago. *It wasn't always like this,* he reminisced.

When he was younger, much younger, everyone in the family had been happy. Everybody got along with each other. They all enjoyed each other. There were long rides through the city and into the country. There were Saturdays and Sundays in the park where Brian and his sister used to swim at the recreation aquatic center. Sometimes they would all sit around and play games at night or talk about school or the weekend to come.

There were those special occasions when relatives and friends came over for birthdays and holidays. It seemed like such a long time ago. It seemed like forever.

And then suddenly, almost overnight, things began to change.

Brian's dad had lost his job at the factory where he was a supervisor. He remembered that day like it was yesterday. His father came home early, threw his jacket down, grabbed a bottle of beer from the garage fridge, and started drinking.

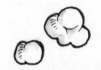

"What's wrong, Marshall?" he had heard his mother ask with a loving, concerned tone in her voice. "What's wrong, dear?"

"They fired me! Can you believe it? They fired me and they're closing down the factory in a couple of weeks. I'm out of a job!" Brian saw the shocked look on his mother's face.

"What are we going to do now, Marshall? What now?"

"I don't know," he snapped as he grabbed another bottle of beer and poured the contents into his mouth. "I don't want to talk about it. Just leave me alone."

He saw his mother cry as he had never seen her cry before. After a while when the beer bottle was almost gone he saw his father weep, too. Brian was shocked. He'd never seen his father cry before. He ran and hid in his bedroom and didn't show his face all night.

No one in the family spoke about what had happened. They all lived together as if nothing had gone wrong or even changed. Days, weeks, and months went by when his father would go out looking for work, come home, and start drinking again. Sometimes, when Brian was in the living room, his father would be drunk and he'd start talking to him.

"You can't trust anybody, Brian. You work your heart and soul out for someone and then they get rid of you. Life's not fair. Remember that Brian. Life's not fair." Brian would listen as his dad mumbled his words.

"Same thing happened to my father. You never knew your grandpa, did ya? He got fired from his job, too, and you know what? It broke his heart and he drank himself to death. You never knew that, but I'm telling you, he drank himself to death. Well, that's not going to happen to me. No sir! The same thing is not going to happen to me that happened to my dad. I'm going to get another job and be better than ever. You wait and see. I'll show them all. I'll be better than ever."

In time, Brian's father did get a job, but something had changed. The family stopped going to the park. They stopped talking, and his mom and dad stopped showing affection toward one another. There were no more hugs like before or playful wrestling matches on the living room floor. His sister started having problems in school, his father never really stopped drinking, and Brian got bigger and bigger.

There were times when the relatives came over, but not as often, and when they did there seemed to always be a fight.

Brian came out of his reverie to the sound of a loud crackle of thunder. Shifting himself on the bed, he put a pillow over his mound of stomach. Hugging the pillow as if he were hugging a teddy bear, he gazed lovingly at Rumps.

After giving up hope for the magical drawer and what it would bring, Rumps had fallen asleep. With one paw crossed over the other, his flabby jaws resting on his paws, he would have no cares until tomorrow.

I envy him, Brian thought. *How wonderful it must be to be a dog or cat or a bird. Free to do whatever you want with no problems or worries. It must be nice to just play and eat.*

He turned his attention back to the ceiling. He remembered the times when he and his big sister were close and she took care of him. He felt protected. He felt like he had someone who was close to him.

"You'd better leave my brother alone!" she'd yell.

"Oh, yeah. What are you going to do about it?"

"You'll see. Push him one more time and you'll see."

"How come you're always sticking up for him?"

"Because he's my brother, that's why. That's what I'm supposed to do." The two kids who had been picking on Brian gave a huff and began walking away. "You're not always going to be around to take care of him, you know," one of them had yelled back.

"Yeah, so you better watch out," the other one added.

"Come on, Brian, let's go home. Don't worry about those stupid guys. If they bother you again, I'll take care of them."

Madison was faster and stronger than anyone in their grammar school. She wasn't about to let anybody pick on her younger brother. She didn't know why they picked on him, anyway. So he wasn't as fast as the rest of the kids and maybe he was just a little on the chubby side. What difference did that make? He was still her brother and she was going to look out for him.

The years they had spent in elementary school together were good times. Sometimes they had played catch or volleyball after school. When they finished playing, they would walk home together hand in hand talking about what they'd done that day and sharing each other's art projects.

But that had changed, too. Unless they were being mean to each other they usually didn't know if the other was alive. Just like the family had stopped spending time together at home, so had Madison and Brian stopped spending time together at school.

As time passed, if there was trouble Madison just ignored it. And as Brian got fatter, she would often join in when the other kids teased him.

After she graduated and went to junior high they never even talked. If they should happen to walk by each other and she was with her friends she would ignore him. The fact was that she didn't want anybody to know that Brian was her brother.

I hate her for that, he thought as he came out of his daydream. *She used to care about me and now she doesn't. My dad used to care about me, but now he's not around much anymore, and when he is around I don't know what to expect, so I'm better off just staying out of his way. I love Mom, but it seems like all she does is complain about my dad and how she wished that she wasn't here. If it weren't for me and Madison she would probably be gone.*

I wish we were like Jeff's family. Everybody is so happy and they have so much fun. I wish we could go back to being the way we were. I wish . . .

Brian began to feel strange. He was up later than usual and he didn't know if he was tired. He thought he was angry, but he didn't know why. His throat was dry and he felt like having a soda. Most of all he was lonely, so very, very lonely. He missed Josh. His eyes began to get wet. He rolled over and opened his stash drawer and grabbed twice as much candy as he had ever taken out before, and then stuffed his mouth until his tears went away.

Brian ripped open a caramel chocolate candy bar and took a huge bite. Once again he stared at Rumps. With a mouth full of candy bar, knowing that the sleeping dog would not hear him he said, "Life's not fair. It's just not fair. Just like Dad always says."

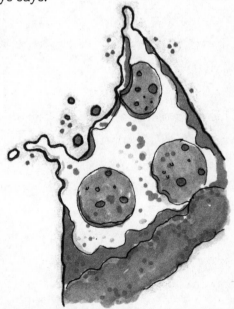

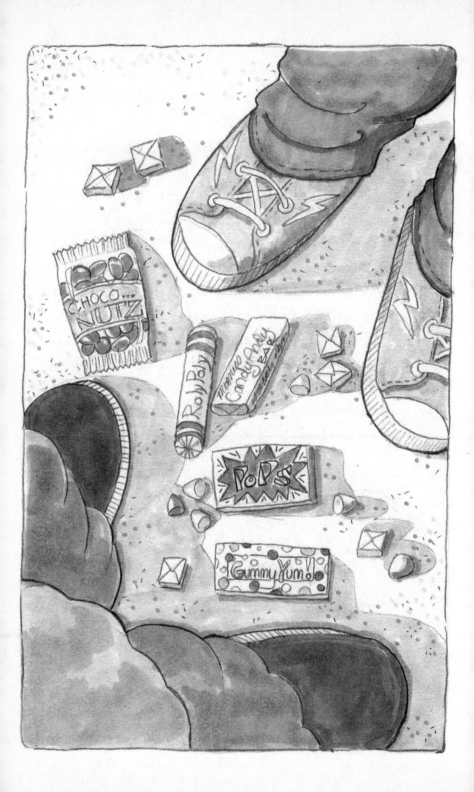

Busted

It's my lucky day, Brian thought as he looked out the window of the school bus. The clock in the middle of the solid brick tower in front of school was staring him straight in the face. The big hand showed Brian that it was fourteen minutes before the Roman numeral twelve. It was exactly 7:46 a.m., which meant that it gave him just enough time to do what he had done so many times before.

Brian hurriedly stepped off the bus, forgetting to say good-bye to Mr. Roberts. Instead of making his usual move toward the school entrance, Brian turned and went in the opposite direction away from school to a destination a block and a half away.

Because there were only fourteen minutes left before class would begin, Brian moved more quickly than he usually did to make it to Rockie's, the school's local candy and junk food shop.

Brian got lucky about once a week, sometimes twice a week. Usually the school bus arrived just minutes before the school's loud, annoying buzzer would go off, giving the command for all students to head to class. Sometimes Mr. Roberts, the bus driver, skillfully maneuvered his way across town and would arrive at school well before class time.

Brian realized that it took more than skill to get the bus to the front of the school well before the buzzer would go off. He had seen luck work to his advantage before. Sometimes the train, which would speed across the city every day, was a few minutes late, allowing the bus to avoid its seven minute wait at the railroad tracks. There were just those days when every street light seemed to magically turn green as the bus would approach. There were other days when the bus didn't make as many stops because there weren't any students waiting for its arrival. If a combination of these lucky events took place, the bus would reach Overton Junior High well before school started.

Brian walked into Rockie's and looked straight up at the clock. "Nine minutes before buzzer time," he mumbled to himself. He shuffled his feet to the aisles that held all the candy treasures. Everything that he had imagined would be there was on the shelves right before his eyes.

Reaching into his pocket, Brian pulled out the money he was carrying. He opened his hand to expose his palm and stared at its contents. He quickly counted two quarters, three nickels, and three pennies. *Not nearly enough for this shopping spree*, he thought. *I should have taken more.*

In the morning just before Brian left for school he usually saw his opening. He'd gotten quite good at slipping back up the stairs to his parents' room and getting the spare change from his dad's pocket. His dad always left his pants draped over the wooden chair against the bedroom window, which made Brian's treasure hunt very easy.

In the years that Brian had learned to go "change fishing," he had never been caught. His dad, who for some reason never emptied his pockets, always left something behind.

Brian could count on a couple of quarters and some other small change in each pocket. Once in a great while a dollar bill would show up, much to Brian's delight.

Brian got an allowance every week, even though he had to remind his parents at times. But they made him save most of it, and what was left he could easily spend in one day after school. So, he just had to get some extra money from somewhere.

He needed the extra money to keep his magic stash drawer full, kind of like the way his mom kept the refrigerator full and his dad kept the liquor cabinet full.

The money he retrieved from his dad's pants pockets usually kept him well supplied. But this morning's fishing expedition revealed little for his efforts.

Brian scanned longingly over the rows of candy. As he did his eyes grew wider, his mouth became moist, and his hands were readied to grab the candies of his choice.

Oh, I've got to have this or I'll just die, and this one's good too, he thought to himself. *And I love this one, too.* In a little more than a minute Brian's hands were grabbing at a half-dozen pieces of candy, most of which he didn't have the money for.

Knowing from the start that his funds would not cover what the cost of the candy would be, he laid out his plan to steal what he wanted.

There were other kids in the store who were buying things as Brian was making his decision. Brian knew that whenever the man working behind the counter used the cash register he had to turn his back away from the candy counter to ring up the sale.

He decided that when the register was being used he would stuff all the candy under his bulky sweatshirt and pick out something he could buy for sixty-eight cents.

Just as Brian looked up, the man behind the counter walked to the register to ring up a sale. Brian quickly stuffed the candy beneath his sweatshirt and grabbed a package of candy-coated peanuts for Rumps.

"Sixty-six cents," Brian read aloud, still standing at the candy counter. At that instant a candy bar fell from his sweatshirt and landed right on his foot. Brian froze. He had stolen candy before, but nothing like this had ever happened.

The man behind the counter turned around and noticed Brian's rigid face.

"Can I help you, son? Any particular thing you're looking for?"

"Uh, um, no thanks. I got it. Oh, here it is." Brian bent over, crushing the candy in his sweatshirt. He picked up the candy bar that was still on his foot and placed both items on the counter in front of the sales clerk.

"Well, son, I'm glad to see you're not buying as much sweet stuff as you usually do. We love the business, but you shouldn't be eating so much of that junk, you know. It's just not healthy for you."

"Yes, sir," Brian said nervously, "I know it. This stuff's not for me anyway. I, uh, got it for the kids at school." The clerk had an "I don't believe you" smirk on his face.

"Good for you, son. You'll lose all that weight eventually."

"Yes, sir. Here, I don't think the kids gave me enough money."

"Well, let's see here. Sixty-six and thirty-nine, that's a dollar and five cents. How much have you got?"

Brian reopened the palm of his hand exposing the money that he had been clutching since he arrived in the store. His palms were all sweaty and the coins easily slipped to the counter.

"Well, son, you've only got sixty-eight cents here. But I'll tell you what I'll do. If you want the one for thirty-nine cents, I'll throw in a couple of pennies."

"Oh, no sir," Brian said sincerely. "I couldn't do that. I'll just take these," pointing to the peanuts.

"See you, son," the clerk said, giving him back the two cents change that was on the counter.

Brian quickly left Rockie's. As he got outside he looked through the store window. The clock now showed three minutes till school was to start.

Brian began a fast-paced walk back to school. He was shaking when he ripped open the package of candy-coated peanuts with his teeth, forgetting that he had bought them for Rumps. He poured the whole package into his mouth. With his chipmunk cheeks bulging with candy he scurried down the block toward school, both hands holding his stomach where his stolen goods were stored.

Moving as quickly as he could, he maneuvered his way to the locker that he had once shared with Josh. He wanted to get rid of his stash of candy and maybe keep one in between the pages of his notebook just in case he needed to munch on something between classes.

He fumbled with the lock, trying to get it to work. Just as the combination was completed and the lock fell open, he felt a slap in the middle of his back.

"Come on, Brian, we're going to be late," Jeff said. As he spoke they both looked down at Brian's feet. Jeff's friendly slap on Brian's back had caused Brian to lose hold of the bundle under his sweatshirt, sending all the candy plummeting to the ground.

"Oh, hi, Jeff. I brought you some candy." Brian said quietly to cover the embarrassment he felt for getting "busted." As the candy-coated peanuts churned in his stomach, Brian swore he would never steal candy from Rockie's again.

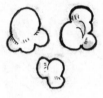

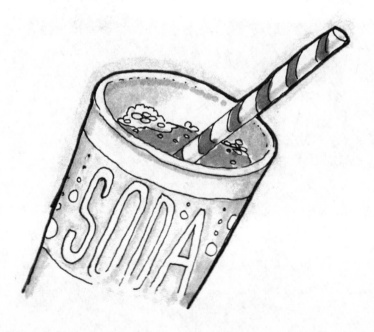

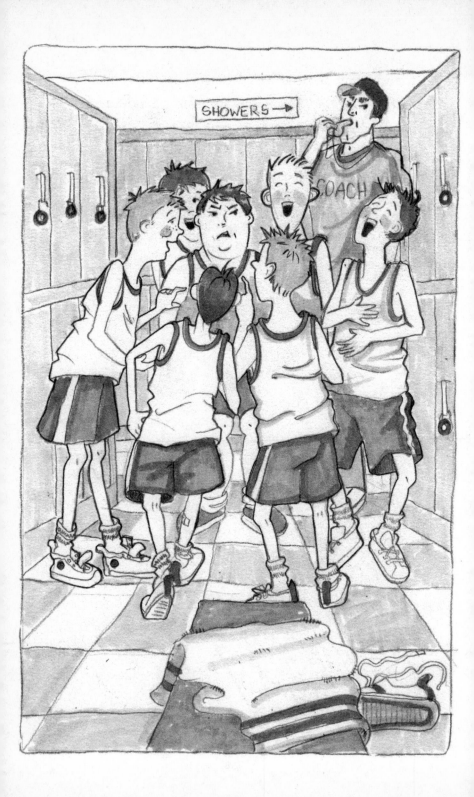

The Day of the Big Exam

Brian was not looking forward to Wednesday morning and what it would bring. He had been dreading this day for weeks. Today was the day for PE exams. He didn't mind history or math or English or any of the other classes. He didn't even mind written tests in PE, but the physical test ran a close second to going to the dentist, which he hated and feared more than anything. In fact, for Brian, PE was like pulling teeth.

He went through his normal routine of getting ready for school. He rummaged through the closet, only to end up with his same old sweatpants and oversized T-shirt. He threw Rumps a few toys and grabbed a before-breakfast snack from the infamous stash drawer by his bed.

Brian trudged into the kitchen, head hung down and hand grasping at his throat.

"What's wrong, Brian?" his mother asked with a concerned tone in her voice as she sat at the table smoking a cigarette and drinking coffee.

"I don't know, Mom," Brian answered, still clutching at his neck. "I think I'm getting a sore throat. I just don't feel good."

"Well, get yourself some breakfast. You'll feel better."

"Okay, but, um, will you write a note to my PE teacher?"

Madison was sitting at the table listening and watching Brian's dramatic antics.

"You've got to be kidding." she exclaimed. "You have just got to be kidding! You're no sicker than the man in the moon. You go through this every time you're going to have a test in PE. Mom, are you going to let him get away with this stuff? If it's not his throat, it's his stomach and if it's not his stomach, it's his foot. He's always faking it to get out of going to PE."

It seemed like Brian's mom was always writing him a note to get out of PE. There was even one time when the school had called her up wanting to speak with her about it. In response to their request she went down to meet with the PE coach.

"As I explained to you, we're very concerned about Brian's attendance in PE."

Fred Larson had been in charge of physical education at Overton Junior High for a number of years. It seemed that there were always students like Brian who bordered on failing PE because they just did not want to participate.

"We feel that Brian needs to become more involved. He's such a superior student in all other areas. Maybe if we could get him involved in one of the team sports or after-school activities he might begin to . . . well, to shape up."

"I don't know. I appreciate your interest in Brian," she said nonchalantly. "But some kids just aren't interested in PE and Brian's one of them. He likes his video games. I wasn't much for PE myself."

Mr. Larson avoided the obvious glance at Brian's mother's obese form sitting before him. He could see that she, too, had not been involved in physical activity for quite some time.

"Well, certainly I understand, but I felt that I should give you my opinion as his PE coach."

Thanking him for his interest, she went on about her business. She gave some consideration to the school's request and even had a long talk with Brian about it. But not more than a week had gone by before Brian complained of another illness and requested a note. His mother had given in and written the note, much to Mr. Larson's frustration.

"Is that true, Brian? Is there a PE test today?" his mother inquired.

"Well, I think so, but my throat really does hurt."

"You big fat liar!" Madison yelled, suddenly standing up from the breakfast table and moving to leave the room. "You're nothing but a big fat fake."

"Madison, you know I don't like it when you call Brian fat," her mother yelled after Madison. "Come back and eat something!" The only response heard was the sound of the slamming front door.

"Brian," she snapped. "Eat your breakfast and march yourself to the bus stop."

"But, what about my note?"

"I'm not writing you a note. Now shut up and finish your breakfast," she said as she stuffed a donut into her mouth.

Brian didn't say another word. He did as he was told. He didn't want to upset his mother any more than he already had.

The first three periods at school seemed to race by, much to Brian's dismay. If he could have reached up and held back the little hand on the clock he would have. But without fail the buzzer sounded at the moment the clock struck eleven.

Brian lumbered his way across the school grounds and into the locker room only to hear the sound of voices yelling, lockers slamming, and towels snapping. At the moment he rounded the corner into the main locker area, a dirty T-shirt hit him smack in the face. The boy who had been intended to receive the flying dirty rag let out a loud laugh.

"Well, I guess you couldn't miss that target, could ya, Billy?"

"Yeah, well, I hadn't expected fat boy to come around the corner," Billy yelled, as he stood on the locker room bench.

Brian pulled the T-shirt from his face, threw it on the floor, and kept on walking, ignoring the comments.

"Hey, Tub-o-lard!" Allen yelled. "Yo, Blubber Butt. You really goin' to take the PE test today? You're never going to pass it."

"Yeah," Billy added. "I don't think Porky has got a chance. It's doomsday for Mister Jumbo." Brian turned around and glared at the two boys.

"Why don't you guys mind your own business?" he said, waving both arms as if to punch them away. Allen began to walk toward him.

"You want to make something of it, Tubby? You want to make me mind my own business?" Allen took his index finger and shoved it into Brian's soft belly.

"You'd better knock it off," Brian snapped.

"You boys have got two minutes to get out on that field," Coach Larson belted out as he marched through the locker room. "Allen, is this your T-shirt on the floor?"

"Yes, Mr. Larson, that's mine."

"Well, I figured that. It's got your name written all over it. Why don't you pick it up, put it on, and get out to the field. Pronto!"

"Yes sir." Allen snatched the T-shirt up on a run, heading for the field.

"Come on, Brian. Let's suit up. I want you out on the field with everyone else."

As Brian opened his locker an odor reeked from inside. He rarely took his gym clothes home to be washed, and knowing that it was nearing the end of the school year he'd decided to let it go an extra two weeks.

The shorts and torn T-shirt with Overton Junior High across the front showed every ripple of his chubby physique. The shorts had fit at the beginning of the school year, so Brian figured they must have shrunk. He had to tear them up each leg a little so that the material wouldn't cut off the circulation in his thighs as he walked. Grabbing an opened bag of jelly beans that he kept in his locker, he threw a handful in his mouth and headed for the field.

"Okay everybody, listen up," Coach Larson commanded as he stood in front of the PE class. "As everybody knows, this is going to be your final grade in PE. I've already graded your multiple choice tests that you took yesterday. Today is the physical exam. Coach Woods is going to assist me since we're breaking off into two groups."

Most of the class was listening intently for their instructions, but Brian was off in another world. Lying flat on the pavement, legs spread apart and arms flung

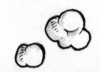

from his side, he gazed into the white marshmallow clouds overhead.

I hate this, I hate this, I hate this, I hate this, he thought over and over. *I don't want to be here. Why do I have to be here? Stupid old PE. I'm never going to be a football player or a track star. Why do I have to do this? Can't they just leave me alone?*

"Brian. Hey, Brian, you want to join the group?" Coach Larson said sarcastically.

Everybody turned around to stare at what looked like a white walrus bathing in the sun. Brian inched his way up onto his elbows and then leaned forward, grunting as he tried to cross his legs Indian style, like everyone else.

"Sorry," he said.

"Okay, let's get started. This half goes with Coach Woods, the rest of you with me."

Billy and Allen ended up with the group that went with Coach Woods. That was a relief to Brian. They had always given him trouble, ever since the school year began. On the other hand, he wasn't real thrilled about being in the group with Coach Larson. He was the tougher of the two coaches and Brian knew it.

He remembered the beginning of the school year when Coach had told everybody about his college days on the football team and how physical education was so important for keeping the body healthy. Brian thought that was a bunch of junk, but he had to admit that the Coach looked like someone he had once seen in a sports magazine.

"All right, first I want everybody to weigh in. Line up in front of the scale and let's get started."

Everybody bustled and shoved to be first in line, except Brian who happily took last place. He couldn't stand for the rest for his classmates to be around while he weighed in. One by one they stepped on the scale.

"Ninety-seven pounds," Coach Larson said, reading the weight on the scale in front of him. "Head out to the track. Next. One hundred-two-and-a-half. Next. Eighty-seven and three quarters." As the line shortened Brian became more uneasy. Soon the line had come to its end.

"Come on, Brian, we haven't got all day. Get up here." Brian stepped on the scale with his leg dangling and the toes of his left foot slightly touching the ground. Brian played this little game with himself whenever he got on the scale. He had hopes that the scale would be more kind that way.

"Brian," Coach said sternly, "both feet on the scale." He responded slowly and when the weights finally settled, Fred Larson read the total to himself. He gazed back at his chart where all the weights of the students were listed from the beginning of the year. He made a quick comparison of Brian's previous weight. After a short hesitation, he asked Brian to step down.

Brian began to head for the field when he felt Coach Larson's firm hand on his shoulder.

"Wait a minute, Brian. Just hold on there. All the other teachers are responsible for teaching you and preparing you for the future. Part of my job is to help you get and stay healthy, but that's not what happened to you in my class. In fact, what has happened is very destructive. You have gained fourteen-and-a-quarter pounds since the beginning of the school year. Tell me, what do you think of that?"

"Well ... I um ... Coach Larson, I haven't been feeling too well and my mom, well, she doesn't like it when I get sick from being in PE."

Fred Larson had well remembered the meeting with Brian's mother. He chose not to respond to Brian's comment.

"Brian, I simply don't understand. You get straight 'A's in all your classes and you even got an 'A' on the written portion in PE. If it wasn't for that 'A' you would get an 'F' instead of a 'D.' Your attendance is terrible, too."

Brian's head was hanging as limply as his arms. He did not want to look the coach in the eye.

"I know you know about health. You know about protein and carbohydrates and cholesterol. Your test tells me that you know how bad sugar is for you and yet you choose to ignore everything that you know. Why, tell me why?"

Brian shrugged his shoulders in a slow motion and lowered them back into place.

"Well, will you at least try to stop eating so much?" Coach Larson asked. "Do you take the bus home from school?"

Brian nodded his lowered head yes.

"Well, how about walking to school or at least take the bus halfway and then walk the other half. That would be very healthy for you and it could help you lose some weight," the coach suggested.

"Yes, sir. I'll try to stop eating so much and I will walk more." Brian knew that it was no trouble to stop overeating. He had done it hundreds of times before. The problem was he had started back just as many times, and each time he did he ate just a little bit more than the time before. He thought about the bus and how he would get out of breath when he walked only three blocks and his house was one mile from the school. He didn't like walking or anything that made him have to work hard.

The physical exam was even more grueling than Brian had thought it would be. He had barely completed three push-ups when the rest of the class had completed their twenty-five.

He was the only one in the class who could not complete the fifty sit-ups and had even struggled at completing sixteen.

Chin-ups were out of the question. He was never able to get beyond grabbing the bar, lifting his heels off the ground, and leaving his toes to support him. But the worst test was yet to come.

"All right, everybody line up in front of the white line. Your last test is going to be one lap around the track. The quicker you complete the lap, the better your grade." They all prepared themselves for the race against time. "Runners, take your mark! Get set! Go!"

The whole class, including Brian, seemed to take a giant step forward at the same time. That was the last moment that Brian would see anything except the backs of his fellow classmates.

He waddled around the track as the rest of the class sprinted out of reach to the finish line. After three minutes had passed with the rest of the class waiting and watching for his completion the shouting and teasing began.

"Hey, Brian, why don't you try riding a turtle? It'd be faster."

"Come on, Tubs, we haven't got all day."

A group of them got together to yell in unison, "Fatty, fatty, two-by-four, couldn't get through the bathroom door."

As Brian reached the last twenty-five feet, one of them ran alongside of him, imitating his waddle and making the sound of a snorting pig. Some of the students didn't participate in the teasing. Although none of them were Brian's size, a few of them were also overweight. Even though they didn't stop the others from the teasing, they each had a sense that the ridicule could just as well have been directed at them.

When Brian stepped over the finish line he fell exhausted onto the grass that bordered the track. The sound of laughter was abruptly interrupted by an angry Coach Larson who stood before them, feet spread apart firmly planted in the ground, and muscular hands gripping his hips.

"I'm ashamed of you. Every last one of you. Who in the world taught you to tease a fellow human being because they are different or because they can't do the same things you can? How rude and mean and inconsiderate."

"Yeah, but he's too fat. He looks stupid." The coach glared at the student.

"So you choose to laugh at him for that? Just because he's different than you? Should I laugh at you because you wear glasses and I don't?" The student who had made the remark hung his head as he pushed his glasses up on the bridge of his nose with his finger.

"And what about you?" pointing to another student. "Should I tease you because your hair is red and no one else in the class has red hair? And you," he said even more firmly. "Can I make fun of you because you wear braces?"

There was an uncomfortable silence as the students sat listening to the reprimand. The only sound that could be heard was Brian gasping for air.

"And how about you? How about if I make fun of you because you're shorter than everybody else or you because you're taller?" He paused again looking over the class as if he were waiting for a reply he knew would never come. "We're all different in this world and each of you is old enough to have learned that by now."

"None of you has the right to treat another human being disrespectfully simply because he or she is different or simply because that person is not like you." Coach Larson hesitated for a moment. "You've made me angry and I'm disappointed in all of you," he scolded. "Everybody hit the showers."

No one spoke as they slowly rose from the ground to their feet and began walking to the locker rooms. Brian moaned as he got to his feet and began walking after the class.

"Brian," the coach said. "I want to tell you one more thing. Being different isn't a bad thing, but being overweight is not healthy. I know you can do better. And I know you can learn how to eat and be healthier."

Brian did not reply. A reply was not needed. He knew in his heart that Coach Larson was right. Entering the locker room, Brian was aware that the silence had made its way inside.

For now there would be no more laughter at Brian's expense. Just for today, the teasing was over.

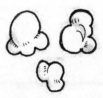

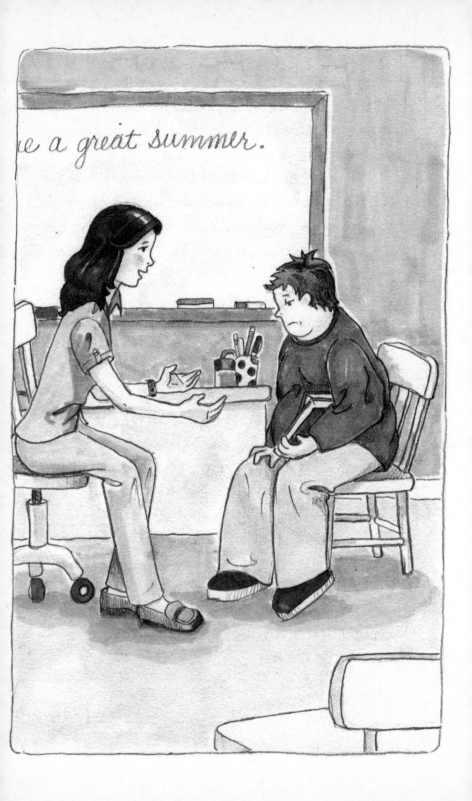

Thank You Ms. Diaz

Ms. Diaz was standing at the blackboard finishing up the last stroke of the letter "R." She had just written a short sentence for her sixth period class when the bell rang. "Have a great summer!" she'd written. A message that she wanted all the children to see before their vacation began. As she turned away from the blackboard to view her class as they began to arrive it was clear to see that she, too, was more than prepared for a wonderful summer vacation. She normally dressed herself in a conservative blouse and bland-colored skirt with shoes to match, but today she allowed herself the pleasure of enjoying the last day of school with the children.

Today she'd chosen a bright purple top with tan jeans. She was sure not to be missed on this final day of school since this was a great departure from her usual outfits.

Sometimes I don't believe it, she thought to herself. *If anyone would have told me that I'd be teaching in the same place for ten years I would have said that person was crazy. I had always thought I would be married with a couple of my own kids instead of taking care of everyone else's.*

But for some reason the thirty-four-year-old Ms. Diaz had just never met anyone to her liking. The closest she had ever come was a young man she had gone to school with, but in their senior year of college they drifted apart and she hadn't seen him since.

Sometimes I think I'll never . . . , her thoughts were quickly interrupted.

"Hi, Ms. Diaz. I mean, hello, Ms. Diaz," Robert said as he came storming into the room.

"Hey, Ms. Diaz," Mark said, following close behind.

"Good afternoon, Ms. Diaz," Sara said with her innocent voice, and one by one they shuffled, pushed, or ran into the classroom.

"Okay, come on, simmer down, simmer down," Ms. Diaz said, clapping her hands. "I know it's the last day of school and you're all excited, but we've still got a few more things to do and then I'm going to let you all go early." A sudden cheer disrupted the calm that Ms. Diaz had asked for.

A paper plane shot its way across the room from the back and two wads of paper struck the ceiling and came plummeting down, one hitting the floor and the other hitting Ms. Diaz right on the tip of her petite nose.

"Who did that?" she snapped. "Come on, who did it?"

The class suddenly went silent, but not one hand was raised, admitting to the heinous crime. She glanced around the now-silent room from left to right and from right to left again. Then suddenly a smile broke out on her face.

"Oh, well," she said, "it is the last day of school." She heard the crack of a cheer breaking. "But if it happens again," she added, one finger pointing to the ceiling, "you're all going to be held after class for thirty minutes, instead of going home early."

Moans and groans sprang out from around the room.

"Okay, let's get started. James."

"Here," he said.

"Robert."

"Here."

"Misha."

"Here."

"Sheila."

"Here."

"Brian. Brian?" She looked up from her roll sheet and at that moment Brian sauntered through the door.

"Here," he said, walking to his seat.

"You're late, Brian," Ms. Diaz pointed out. "Do you have an excuse?"

"Yes, Ms. Diaz. I was . . ."

"He was finishing his third lunch," Kyle uttered. The whole class broke out in laughter.

"That's enough. Brian, just sit down. I'll talk to you after class."

Ms. Diaz finished taking the roll and with everybody in attendance she began her last-day-at-school speech. The same speech she made every year, with one big exception.

". . . and finally, I want to tell you all something before we get to our last assignment. I've decided that I'm not going to come back next year. I've been teaching children just like you for ten years now. So, I've decided to do something a little different. For my summer, I'm going to travel all over the country, and when the summer is over I'm going to go back to school and get what's called a master's degree."

"Yuck!" Neil screamed. "Go back to school. I'd never go back. I can't wait to get out. What are you going back to school for?"

"Well, with more education I can do different things, and life has lots of challenges to it. So I want to experience some of them."

"Will we ever see you again?" Sandra asked.

"Sure. I'm going to come back and visit you after the summer. If I didn't, I'd miss you all."

She got a few more questions and when they were all answered, Ms. Diaz walked to the blackboard and began to write. All eyes in the classroom watched as she wrote, "What I'm going to do on my summer vacation." When she was done she put down her chalk and turned to the class.

"Okay, I want you all to get out a pencil and paper and tell me what you're going to do for your vacation."

"Do we have to?" Jamie moaned.

"If you want to get out of here early," she said without a pause.

The sound of shuffling papers and pencils against the desktops came as soon as she finished her sentence. "I'm going to give you twenty minutes, and when you're done you may put your paper on the corner of my desk and start your summer vacation."

Ms. Diaz stood at the corner of her desk for a moment while the children began to write. After about thirty seconds, when they had settled into their project she maneuvered her way around her desk and into her chair of ten years. She clasped her hands in front of her, leaned into the back of her chair, both feet firmly on the floor and began to gaze around the room.

My goodness, she thought. *I'm going to miss you, old friend. Your four walls have been company to me for the best one third of my life. It's going to seem strange to be without you.* She giggled at herself for giving the room the qualities of a person and quickly turned her thoughts to the children in front of her.

For the last ten years the same students had come and gone from her class: a Thomas, Katie, Amanda, Allen, Tony. The list of names went on. She merely had to attach a different face to an already-memorized list of names. With each face she saw a different personality. Some happy, some sad. But all in all, the years had supplied her with some of her favorite memories.

He's going to become a doctor, she thought. *That one in the corner of the room, I think she'll be a lawyer. He's destined to go into sports. I can barely keep him in his seat when there's a game to be played after school. I'm not sure about that one, but she's going to be something special.* And as her thoughts about the children roamed from one to the next, she finally reached Brian and her mind froze.

Each year there was at least one Brian in her class. And each year her heart went out to that child. Some years it was a boy and some years it was a girl. But no matter who the particular child was, she felt that child's pain.

Why is Brian so fat? she asked herself. And with the question came the answer. As she stared at Brian, her own childhood came rushing back.

"Nancy! Nancy Diaz. Get in this house this minute. Your father is going to be home and he wants his dinner on the table the moment he gets in. You didn't get that dress dirty, did you? You'll get a beating for sure. Did you do your homework? I bet you didn't do your homework. Why can't you be more like your brother? He always does so well in school. Get your hands out of the cookie jar. If I've told you once I've told you a thousand times. No more cookies! Bet you spent your lunch money on that junk food again. Nancy, you're getting as big as a house. As it is you can only wear two dresses and your father is not about to give me any more money to buy you new clothes. So you better just cut it out. What the heck am I going to do with you? You keep it up and you're going to look just like me."

A vision of her mother followed her memory. Short and fat with skin under her arms that hung loosely, two chins that were growing into a third, and thighs that could not be distinguished from an already enormous waist.

A tear welled up in her eye as she began to remember the years of pain, ridicule, and harassment she had received from her family and classmates. Not a day had gone by that she had not endured one comment or another about her size.

"You'd be such a pretty little girl if you'd lose some weight."

"Have you tried this diet? It worked for me."

"Try wearing darker clothes. It always seems to hide everything."

She remembered year after year of promising not to take another bite and year after year of having one more candy bar, one more piece of cake, and one more scoop of ice cream.

But then, when there seemed to be no hope, she met someone who changed her life. She met someone who was willing to let her feel. To be loved for who she was and express herself in any way she wanted. She remembered the hours of pain and feelings that she had never felt in her life before and the unconditional love that took place hour after hour, day after day, and month after month.

In time, a long time, she remembered how the pounds began to peel off her obese body. She accepted her past for what it was. She chose not to hate, but rather to love herself. She chose to live life as it was intended to be lived, for herself, with all the happiness and health that she deserved.

"Teacher. Teacher. Ms. Diaz." She suddenly snapped her head back and blinked her eyes as she woke from her trance. "Ms. Diaz, have a wonderful summer. My mom said to tell you thanks for helping me with my spelling."

"You're welcome, Ryan. You have a great summer, too."

One by one the students brought their papers to the corner of her desk, left them where they were instructed to, and said their good-byes. There were a few students left when Brian reached the desk.

"Sorry I was late, Ms. Diaz. I got uh, um, uh . . . hung up."

"Brian, would you please wait for the other students to leave? I'd like to talk to you after class for a few minutes."

"Oh, c'mon, Ms. Diaz. Honest, I couldn't help it."

"Brian, please sit down at your desk."

Brian shuffled his feet all the way back to his desk, plopped down in his chair, and dug both elbows into the desktop as he cradled his chin in the palms of his hands. With a grumpy expression on his face he waited for the others to finish.

A few minutes had passed before the rest of the students had completed their tasks and said their good-byes.

With the room now empty except for Brian and herself, Ms. Diaz made a decision to pass the gift of awareness that she had received on to Brian, hoping that he could understand.

"Brian, why don't you come up here and sit down?" She pointed to the chair that was immediately to the left of her desk. She'd used the chair many times before to reprimand students, to help them with their homework, or to find out why they hadn't completed it.

But this time was going to be very different. As Brian was walking up the aisle of desks that bordered him on both sides, she took her old wooden desk chair from around the back and brought it in front so that she could speak to Brian without any barriers between them.

"Ms. Diaz," he groaned. "I'm sorry I was late, but this is the last day of class. Can't I go home early today with the rest of the kids?"

"Brian," she said with a warm smile on her face, "I'm not keeping you after class to punish you. I was just hoping that we could spend a little time talking. You know you're the best student I have."

"Yeah," he exclaimed, "I got all 'A's again except for that stupid 'D' in PE."

"Oh. How do you feel about that?" she asked with an upbeat tone in her voice. "How does it make you feel?"

"I think PE is dumb. I think you shouldn't have to go if you don't want to."

"Yes. But how does it make you *feel*, Brian?"

"I think it's boring."

"Brian, listen to me," she said warmly, extending an arm out and touching his chubby knee with the deepest compassion. "Try to tell me how it makes you feel inside in your stomach, in your heart."

Brian froze at the touch of her hand and the sound of her words. *I wish she wouldn't touch me*, he said to himself. *I always feel so strange when people touch me. Mom and Dad don't touch me, why does anyone else have to?*

Ms. Diaz sensed his uneasiness and removed her hand.

"Brian, what are you feeling?"

"I don't know. It doesn't make me feel like anything. I don't ever really feel anything. I just kind of ignore it."

"Well," she said with a long hesitation in her voice. "How do you feel when the kids make fun of you and call you mean names or when you don't get to go to the parties or play sports? How does that make you feel?"

"I don't know," Brian said, looking away from her, staring off into the corner of the room. "It's just dumb. It's just boring. I don't care."

She watched him as he stared into the corner of the room, a glazed look in his eye. *How do I tell him?* she thought. *How do I tell him that he must learn how to feel, to enjoy the magical gift of life that he has been given.* She paused for what seemed to be an eternity to Brian.

She finally broke the silence.

"When I was your age, Brian, I was big, too. The truth is I was fat. I hated PE. I never got invited to the parties and the kids made fun of me. And you know what?" Brian was now staring at her, watching her lips as she spoke.

"I was lonely, very, very lonely. It bothered me and my feelings got hurt. Rather than tell people how I felt I would just sit and eat, sometimes at school, sometimes at home, or wherever I was. It wasn't until I learned to tell people how I felt that I began to feel good about myself."

"But the kids make fun of me," he blurted out. "They tease me. They don't like me because I'm fat. I don't care. They're all boring. Whatever."

"Brian, tell them how you feel. Tell them they're hurting your feelings."

Brian began to shake. *I don't want to feel,* he thought. *I don't care.*

"Were you really fat, Ms. Diaz?" Brian said, knowing that he was cutting off his own feelings with the question. "Fat just like me?"

Her body relaxed and she sighed. *I almost got to him,* she thought. *I almost reached him.*

"Yes, Brian, I was fat just like you. Looking back, I realize how much I missed—all the times that I would have had playing and going out to parties and just having a plain old good time. Brian, I know this is difficult for you to understand, but try to listen to what I'm saying. Some people use food to hide their feelings and others use alcohol or other drugs or cigarettes to do the same thing." Brian's eyes widened. He felt like his eyes were going to pop out of his head.

"My dad drinks. My dad drinks a lot of beer. He never talks to me. My mom smokes a lot of cigarettes and she is always eating." *Boy,* Brian said to himself, *sure never thought I would be telling anyone about my family secrets.*

"Some people don't want to *feel* their feelings, so they just work all the time or they never sit still."

Brian didn't think that his eyes could get any wider.

"My dad and sister do that. My sister never sits still!" he exclaimed throwing his arms into the air. "And she's thin, real, real thin and my dad works a lot of hours."

"Being too fat or too thin, Brian, is the same thing. Both can come from not dealing with feelings."

"But Ms. Diaz, I don't understand. How can I feel these things if I've never felt them before?" Brian began to think about the secrets he was expected to keep, then he began to *feel* the secrets that he was expected to keep. He could feel the tears welling up.

Ms. Diaz looked at Brian with deep compassion in her eyes and leaned over and squeezed his hand. Brian took a deep breath and then began to sob. She held his hand in silence and let him cry. She knew how important crying was and let him continue until she felt he could hear her again. As his sobs slowed down, she began to speak.

"If someone hurts you, tell that person what you feel. If someone says something that bothers you, tell that person what you feel, *not* what you think. And Brian, most importantly, and as difficult as it might be, try not to eat when you're feeling something even if you don't know what you are feeling."

"I don't understand," he said still crying slightly. "I just don't understand."

She let go of his hand and looked directly at him.

"I know it's difficult to understand, but promise me you'll try. Promise me that you will talk and tell people how you feel, okay?"

"Okay, Ms. Diaz, I'll try," Brian said, taking the palms of his plump hands and wiping the tears from his eyes.

She gave him a quick smile as he turned and walked to the door. Before leaving the classroom to start his summer vacation, Brian turned and looked at his teacher who was standing at the corner of her desk.

"Thank you, Ms. Diaz. I'll miss you. I wish you weren't leaving."

"I'll miss you, too," she replied, but he didn't hear her words. He had left before she had spoken.

Ms. Diaz walked to the door and closed it tightly. Flipping the lock with one hand and turning off the light with the other she walked back to her desk. Positioning her desk chair back in its place she sat down, placed her arms and hands palm down on the desk one hand over the other, lowered her head, and began to weep. She wept for Brian and what he must go through to get in touch with his feelings in order to have a happy life and lose weight. She wept for the pain she had gone through and the childhood she had missed.

When she was done she picked up a box of already packed belongings and carried the ten years worth of memories out of the classroom.

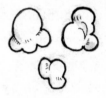

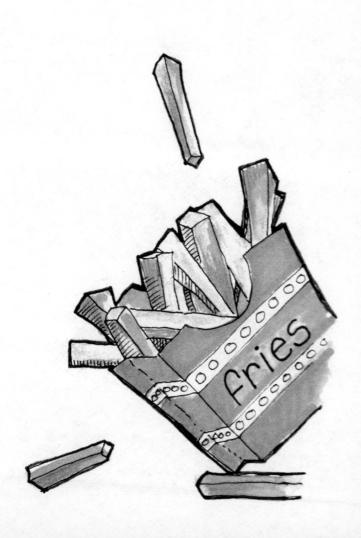

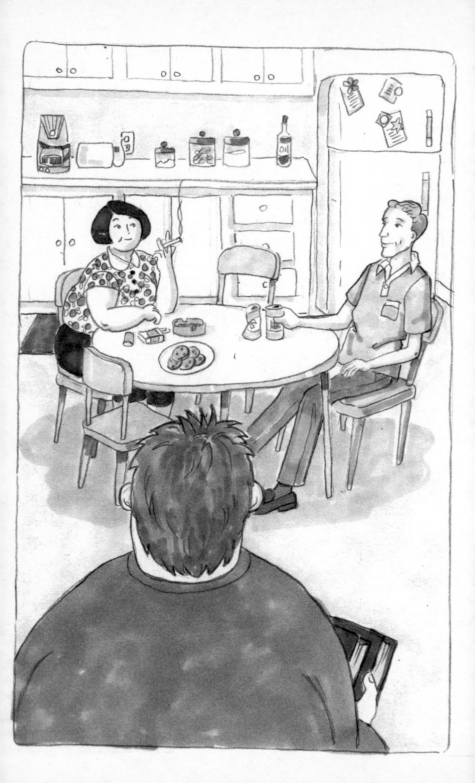

Epilogue

Brian rounded the corner of the block that led to his house. He had decided not to take the bus all the way. So five stops before his usual stop he got off the bus and began to walk the rest of the eleven blocks to his home. As he walked, he reflected on what his teacher had told him.

In the driveway of his home sat his father's two-year-old blue Chrysler. Brian remembered overhearing his dad tell his mother that he would be home early today.

Brian walked up the brick pathway, gripped the door handle tightly, opened the door, took one step, and then he was in the house. Standing taller than he'd ever stood before, he said with a strong voice so that he could be heard throughout the house, "Mom! Dad! I'm home. I really want to talk with both of you. I need to tell you how I feel."

Activity Guide and Discussion Questions

Chapter One: Almost All "A"s

1. What do you think about Brian? Do you like him? Why or why not?

2. What do you think of Brian's family?

3. Do you know anyone like Brian? Are there any ways that you are like Brian?

4. Brian's mom always gave Brian a reward of going out to eat for getting good grades in school; is this a healthy or unhealthy reward?

5. How do you think Brian felt when his father didn't want to look at his report card?

Chapter Two: What's for Dinner?

1. Brian eats snacks between meals. Is a cupcake a healthy between-meal snack? What would be a healthy snack?

2. Do you think it was appropriate for Brian's mom to say the things she said about Brian's dad to Brian? Does she sound like a happy person?

3. How do you think that the comments Brian's dad made about Brian's weight made Brian feel bad? How would comments like that make you feel?

4. Does anyone make mean comments to you? What are those comments? How do they make you feel? How do you respond to those comments?

Chapter Three: The Stash Drawer

1. Why do you think Brian feels like he is different from the other kids in school?

2. Brian is thinking about how the kids at school tease him and is just about to say how he feels about it when his sister interrupts his thoughts. What do you think he was going to say?

3. What does Brian keep in his stash drawer? Why does he call it his stash drawer?

4. Why do you think Brian hid all the candy wrappers?

Chapter Four: Trouble

1. Why didn't Brian's dad go with the family on Brian's special day?

2. Do you know anyone like Brian's friend Josh? Why do you think Josh had problems getting his homework done on time?

3. What was the fight between Josh and Kyle about?

4. Do you get in fights in school? Who starts them, you or someone else?

5. Why do you think the other kids just stood around and cheered the fight on between Josh and Kyle? Have you been a bystander to a fight? What did you do? How could you help break up a fight?

Chapter Five: There's a New Kid in Town

1. Why do you think Josh started the fire at school?

2. How do you think Jeff felt about going to a new school in a new city and state?

3. Why do you think Ms. Diaz asked Brian to show Jeff around the school?

4. What was the difference between Brian's lunch and Jeff's lunch?

5. Why was Brian so excited about going to Jeff's house for dinner?

Chapter Six: If It's Not One Thing, It's Another

1. Have you heard the saying, "If it's not one thing, it's another"? What does it mean?

2. Why was Brian a half hour late for dinner at Jeff's house? Is it okay to be late to places?

3. Why would Brian say that his pants and clothes had shrunk? Do you think he really believed that his clothes had shrunk?

4. Brian's dad had promised to take him to Jeff's house; why did he go back on his promise? How do you feel when someone promises to do something for you and then he or she doesn't?

5. Do you keep your promises?

Chapter Seven: Meet the Armstongs

1. Why did Brian tell lies to Jeff and his family about being late and other things?

2. Why was Brian expecting more food and different food for dinner at the Armstrongs?

3. Would you say that Mrs. Armstrong cooked a healthy meal? Why was it healthy?

4. Brian wasn't anxious to get home. What do you think was waiting for Brian when he returned home from Jeff's house?

Chapter Eight: Yesterday and Today

1. Brian was so excited about his dinner with Jeff, but when he came home his mother only wanted to talk about how mad she was at Brian's dad. How do you think that made Brian feel?

2. Brian's mom made him promise he would keep the family secrets. What were the family secrets and why would his mother want Brian to keep these secrets?

3. Brian's father says that "Life's not fair." What does that mean to you?

4. Brian and his sister used to be so close. What do you think happened to make them argue with each other all of the time?

5. Brian felt sad and started to cry, but as soon as he ate a bite of candy his tears went away. Why do you think that happened?

Chapter Nine: Busted

1. Brian took money from his dad's pants pocket. Would you call this stealing?

2. Why do you think Brian got so excited when he was looking at the candy in the store?

3. Why do you think Brian lied to the store owner about buying the candy for other kids?

4. What do you think about Brian stealing the candy?

5. Have you ever stolen anything? Why do you think you did it?

Chapter Ten: The Day of the Big Exam

1. Why did Brian fake being sick? Have you ever said you were sick when you weren't just to get out of doing something?

2. What do you think about Brian's mom always writing him excuses to get out of PE?

3. Some of the other boys in the PE class called Brian mean names. Why do you think they called him those names? How do you think Brian felt when he was called those names?

4. Have you ever been called mean names? Have you ever teased someone else by calling them mean names? Would you call this bullying?

5. How did you feel about Coach Larson's lecture on being different?

Chapter Eleven: Thank You Ms. Diaz

1. Why did Ms. Diaz want to talk with Brian alone after class?

2. What is the difference between a thought and a feeling?

3. Why do you think Ms. Diaz felt like she could relate to Brian?

4. What did Ms. Diaz want Brian to do if someone said something that hurt his feelings?

5. Why did Ms. Diaz cry after Brian left?

Epilogue

1. What do you think Brian said to his family?

2. Do you think that they listened to him?

3. Before this, Brian didn't share his feelings with anyone. Do you share your feelings? With whom?

4. What could Brian do to cope with his father's drinking? His mother's eating and smoking? His sister's constant put-downs?

5. Why do you think Brian is so fat? What could Brian do to lose weight?

Describe what you think are healthy foods for the following meals:

Breakfast

_____

_____

Lunch

_____

_____

Dinner

_____

_____

Describe what you think a healthy snack would be. Give three examples.

Discuss what you think healthy activities are. Give three examples.

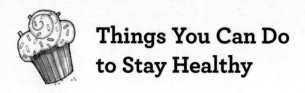

Things You Can Do
to Stay Healthy

Eat healthy foods like

- Fruits and vegetables. Remember the more colorful the fruit or vegetable, the more vitamins and nutritional value it has.

- Fish and chicken

- Beans and nuts

- Whole-wheat brown bread

- Low-fat dairy products, such as milk, cheese, yogurt

Instead of . . .

- Ice cream, eat frozen yogurt or sherbet

- White bread, eat whole wheat

- Potato chips, eat carrot sticks or veggie chips

- Soda, drink water, fruit and vegetable juice, or flavored mineral water

- Sugar-coated cereal, eat cereal with natural sugars added or no sugar at all. Add raisins or fruit to make it sweet.

- Hamburgers and hot dogs, eat turkey or veggie burgers/dogs

Do healthy things like

- Skateboarding
- Walking with friends
- Soccer
- Basketball
- Dancing
- Jump rope
- Helping to clean around the house or yard

- Swimming
- Football
- Baseball
- Riding your bike
- Karate
- Wii interactive video games

Don't do too much of these things

- Play video games
- Watch TV
- Eat in front of the TV
- Ride in the car if you can walk or ride your bike instead

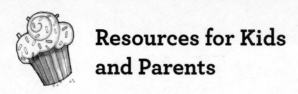

Resources for Kids and Parents

Websites for healthy meal/food/menus/recipes/snacks

www.letsmove.gov

www.HealthierGeneration.org

www.kaboose.com

www.FruitsAndVeggiesMoreMatters.org

www.nickjr.com/recipes/index.jhtml

Websites on obesity and children/kids

www.letsmove.gov

www.kidshealth.org

www.nlm.nih.gov/medlineplus/obesityinchildren.html

www.cdc.gov/healthyyouth/obesity/facts.htm

Websites for exercises for children/kids

www.letsmove.gov

www.exerciseforkids.com

www.keepkidshealthy.com

www.kidshealth.org